The

Food god

Food's connection to our Creator, our community, and our health

Trent Holbert BA, CPT, SNS

Forward by
Dr. Gus Vickery MD

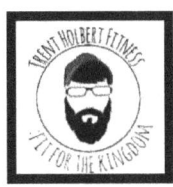

www.trentholbertfitness.com

Copyright © 2020 The Food god

All rights reserved. This book or any portion thereof may not be reproduced or used in any manner whatsoever without the express written permission of the publisher except for the use of brief quotations in a book review.

Printed in the United States of America
First Printing, 2020

ISBN 9781734618303

Trent Holbert Fitness LLC
Black Mountain, NC 28711

www.trentholbertftness.com

Unless otherwise noted, all Scripture quotations are taken from the Holman Christian Standard Bible®, Used by Permission HCSB ©1999,2000,2002,2003,2009 Holman Bible Publishers. Holman Christian Standard Bible®, Holman CSB®, and HCSB® are federally registered trademarks of Holman Bible Publishers.

Contents

Forward	Page 5
Preface	Page 9
Introduction	Page 11

Part One-What's the Point?

Chapter 1: My Story (Part 1-Before)	Page 15
Chapter 2: The Beginning Plate (Food's Role in Establishing a Relationship With God and His People)	Page 37
Chapter 3: The Broken Plate (How Man's Appetite Has Disconnected Him From God)	Page 43
Chapter 4: The Blessed Plate (How Food Connects to God)	Page 47
Chapter 5: The Believer's Plate (How Christians Should Approach Food)	Page 61
Chapter 6: My Story (Part 2-After)	Page 111

Part Two

Recipes	Page 131
Frequently Asked Questions	Page 139
Acknowledgments	Page 149
References	Page 151

Forward

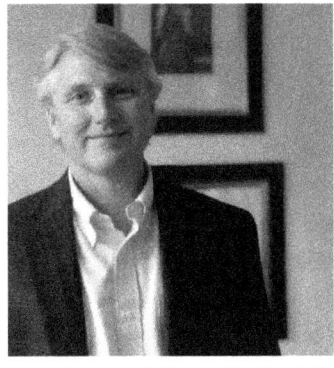

It is my great privilege to write a foreword on behalf of my friend and fellow health professional Trent Holbert. I first met Trent over a year ago. A mutual acquaintance emailed me and suggested I might want to meet this young pastor who is also an expert in nutrition and fitness who had moved into my area. This introduction came at a time that I was incredibly busy with my primary responsibilities. Although I enjoy meeting people, I didn't really feel like I had time to cultivate new relationships given the many responsibilities I was managing. Nonetheless, I was intrigued about the combination of a pastor and an expert in human health, and therefore, I agreed to an afternoon meeting. How grateful I am that I did. My life has been enriched and blessed by my relationship with Trent. He has not only become a strong spiritual mentor for me, he has become one of my best friends.

For years, God had been placing on my heart a desire to share the truth of human health with all people, but especially His church. As a physician whose passion is to study the design of the mind and the body and to cultivate an understanding of what is necessary to optimize our health for the purposes of living at our full potential, I had a strong interest in seeing God's people understand and apply this truth. I saw that many people in the church, who were very committed to living in accordance with God's truth, had become victims of our modern-day food culture that has contributed to our epidemic obesity and metabolic diseases. While we were aware of the destructive potential of many of the sources of addiction in our modern society, we somehow failed to perceive how food itself had become a source of addiction. Many individuals with good intent and with a sincere desire to guard their lives against destructive elements still found themselves with the symptoms of poor health influenced by unhealthy approaches to eating.

Trent and I have shared many long walks in the woods discussing our faith, our understanding of human health, nutrition, physical fitness, and how we could share a message with God's people of hope and healing. Trent is so passionate about the gospel. He also understands that we live our lives within bodies that were designed by a loving creator. When we honor the truth of this design, we have the opportunity to experience healing, freedom from disease, and the ability to experience our full potential. However, in order for this to happen, we must become serious about the information we provide our body. Food is one of the most important sources of information for our body. We have treated food as nothing more than a source of calories. Food is so much more than calories. Food is sustenance. Food provides the energy we need for life. Food provides nutrients, fiber, and energy.

We live in a time that so many people are overfed but undernourished. In order for God's people to experience the fullness of health that is their birthright, we must cultivate a correct understanding of what food is for us. It is pleasure, it is comfort, it is an opportunity to build community and strengthen family relationships, but it is primarily the source of health for our bodies. Modern day foods have become a source of calories with minimal nutrients. Modern day foods have been purposely manipulated to trigger overeating and other dysfunctional eating behaviors. Modern day foods often contain elements that, rather than supporting our health, contribute to disease. Trent understands this, and it is his deep desire to communicate the truth about food and its influence on health to all people and especially God's people.

When I met Trent, I was so encouraged to have met a pastor who deeply understood the importance of proper stewardship of the body. Trent does not only talk the talk; he walks the walk. He and his family were obedient to give away their possessions and travel to a new community where God had sent them. I have observed as God has used him powerfully for the building of the kingdom and supporting the health of those he influences. A church has formed around him and people's lives are being changed. He's become a global ambassador for an organization that has learned how to use the concepts of health and fitness to spread the gospel and build the kingdom of God. It is so clear to me that God is powerfully using this humble pastor who has such a strong heart for his fellow human beings. Trent has a wisdom that has been forged through deep study and real experience. His work is truthful and powerful.

I hope this book spreads far and wide and influences many. As God's people embrace these truths and apply them to their lives, we will become the best examples of what it means to honor this precious gift of life that God has given us. Finally, I want the reader to know that Trent is a gracious individual and does not possess a spirit of judgment towards others. He understands how challenging these truths can be. He understands how many of the patterns of our lives often develop before we were at ages of conscious choice. We do judge systems that would manipulate our sources of sustenance in a way that harms individuals for the purposes of making more money. We judge these systems, but not the individuals who've been victimized. However, it will be up to us to honor these truths, accept the challenge of change, and encourage all of God's people on this journey of living our healthiest lives. Thank you, Trent, for your friendship, your wisdom, and your courage to always speak the truth.

Gus Vickery, MD

Preface

I don't want to dictate how you read this book. The reason you picked it up in the first place is as unique as your own needs. Some people will connect with my personal story of struggles and how I overcame them. You may only need to read the beginning and the end. You will have the ability to connect to my heart and empathize with a fellow human being that has discovered a better way to live through faith and holistic living.

You may be on your own spiritual journey and have an appreciation for food. You may dig into the middle portion of this book and use it as your own devotional to help understand the deep connectedness we can have with our Heavenly Father through a healthier connection to the food that He has provided.

Or, maybe you are a science and health nerd like me. I have enjoyed connecting theological truths to the science aspects of nutrition and biology, human physiology, and herbalism. Whether you align yourself closely with Western medicine or feel more comfortable with alternative natural means of health (or a mixture of the two), you can use this book as a nutritional health book. I really wanted to write this book in such a way that would be used to connect your body, mind, and soul to a better life!

Enjoy!

Introduction

"One cannot think well, love well, sleep well, if one has not dined well."

— Virginia Woolf, *A Room of One's Own*

When was your last meal? A few hours ago? A few moments ago? If you are on an average eating schedule of eating 3-5 meals a day, then while you read these words, you would have eaten already today and/or are getting ready to eat again. Food is usually either a recent thought (past tense) or an imminent thought (near future tense). Some days I go to bed thinking about my next lunch! My week and all my appointments and meetings are usually scheduled around dining and food. Morning coffee meetups at the local café, or a luncheon meeting, or hosting friends for dinner; the dining table IS my office. I even plan my road trips around what restaurants are located near my appointments. My rationale says, "If I go 'this' way, then I can stop and eat at 'such and such' restaurant."

Can we downplay the importance of food in our culture and in our lives? Hardly! The title of this book has already stood out to you. Food god? Perhaps the two most basic tenants of life can be simplified to 'connect with our Creator' and 'eat food'. Well, think about it. As soon as oxygen found its way into our lungs and that first gurgling scream burst forth from our newborn larynx, we were ushered to our mother's breast for our first meal; the first of hundreds of thousands of meals over the course of a lifetime. Within seconds of life, we are eating. Within seconds of eating, our brains sense the release of dopamine, the 'feel good' hormone...teaching us that good food elicits good feelings.

Human beings are created to connect to their Creator and to eat. Without one, there is spiritual death. Without the other, there is physical death. I contend, however, that the latter tends to be more prevalent of a desire from the beginning of life and often more than not, throughout the remainder of life. How many times have you thought about eating today? How many times have you thought about God today? Nature itself teaches us that to live, to survive, we MUST eat. It is so much a part of our being that our entire digestive system runs on innate intelligence. Meaning, you don't have to actually think about sending hunger signals to your brain. The hormone Leptin does that. You don't have to think about breaking down and dispersing food's nutrients, vitamins, and minerals to the appropriate places in the body. We don't even have to think about getting rid of the waste. All we have to think about is when, what, and how much we eat. But then, we seem to be thinking about that A LOT!

This book is not meant to demonize food or cause a sense of guilt for enjoying it. As I've mentioned, food is natural and needed in order to survive. My soapbox on the subject is to show you that food often becomes more important in our lives than the One who created it. Our desires and passions revolving around food, diet, and dining tend to overshadow God's will and purpose for our lives. The results could send us crashing into bad physical health, lack of ability to follow through with God's instructions, sin, or a disconnected relationship with Him. Food plays an important role in our life for survival, obviously, but also in effectively connecting to the world around us through the relationships with friends and family. You will see in the following chapters, how food will play an enormous role in your spiritual survival, as well as connecting to the world around you in such a healthy way. You are either giving in to an appetite of destructions or thriving with a hunger for righteousness.

Also, it is my attempt to examine the keys to total health through the food that we eat. I want to show you that food is intended to be something that brings us closer to God in relationship. Food has an intended spiritual influence over your health. It doesn't stop there. As a holistic health coach, I want to show you that our attitudes toward food, the quality of food, and our diets play a huge role in mental emotional, and of course, physical health. Imagine, the ability to transform your whole being, simply by transforming your dinner plate.

Part 1: What's The Point?

Chapter 1

My Story, Part 1-Before

Shattered, broken, depressed, and in full-time ministry. This was my life at one point. How did I get here?

Who concerns themselves with health and eating right when they're a kid? I think I was pretty normal in the sense that I ate a standard American diet and was a picky eater growing up. I was a farm boy, raised to work hard. As a teenager, my life consisted of long days of physically demanding labor, fueled by pizza, French fries, and fast food. Somehow, I kept up. Most of us do during those young years of high metabolism and surging hormones. By my senior year of high school, I was 5'9" and 166 pounds of lean muscle that was built by carrying and stacking hay bales all summer. There was little to no down time. When I wasn't working on the farm, I was working as a stock boy at a local grocery store, lugging boxes of canned goods and crates of produce. Any free time I had was lived outside playing sandlot baseball, riding bikes, or running the hills and hollows with my friends.

I had "farm" strength. I never went to a gym. That wasn't an opportunity afforded to me, living in a small rural town of north-central Kentucky. That doesn't mean that I didn't have a gym. My dad was legendary in our community. His feats of strength performed for his friends growing up created a sense of pride in him that was destined to be passed down to his two boys. We often heard stories of him picking up 100 lb. sacks of potatoes with his teeth, or leg pressing the back of a cultivating tractor off the ground. My older brother and I were groomed for strength. With every story that we heard of our dad's legendary strength, we felt a sense of heritage, that we too, would build such a legacy. In our side yard, my dad had built a custom-made playground consisting of monkey bars and pull-up rigs. In our barn hung a punching bag. It was to his delight to watch his sons workout, often stepping in to add coaching. I can remember hanging from a barn tier, suspended by my arms, while my dad shadow boxed my stomach in order to build core strength. It was a growing desire to prove my worth through my work ethic and strength to my father.

Our farm was also a strength gym. Along with my grandparents, aunts and uncles, we raised large acreage crops of tobacco and hay, as well as vegetable gardens. There was never any of the work that I actually liked. It was hard work! The older I got, the harder the work became. On a miserably hot June-August afternoon you would find us hauling square hay bales from the field to the barn. As the tractor and wagon traversed across the field, one or two of us would be atop the wagon, stacking bales as another two or three would carry them to load. We switched off regularly. Hay bales would range in weight from fifty to eighty pounds, depending on which uncle baled it that go around. It was hardest working for my uncle Jim, who liked to bale them heavy and tight. In almost an act of spite, I reveled in the ability to carry one bale in each hand to the wagon. "I'll show him how strong I am.", I thought. Guys in the 'globo' gyms think they know what farmer carries are, ha! We knew what a farmer carry was!

On days that there wasn't anything pressing, or perhaps for reasons of corporal punishment, we spent busting and hauling field stone to the hollow. Our fields were littered with Kentucky Limestone, a heavy, dense stone that is not soft to the touch. They had to be removed. Some stones weighing several hundred pounds, some immovable, needed to be busted up into smaller pieces with a sledgehammer and carried or stacked on a wagon. Kentucky is known for its vast limestone deposits. As you drive across the Bluegrass region, you will see many remnants of the old stone fence, running for miles along the highways, built by Scottish stonemasons. We could've built castles with the amount of stones that we spent time busting with sledgehammers and piling up.

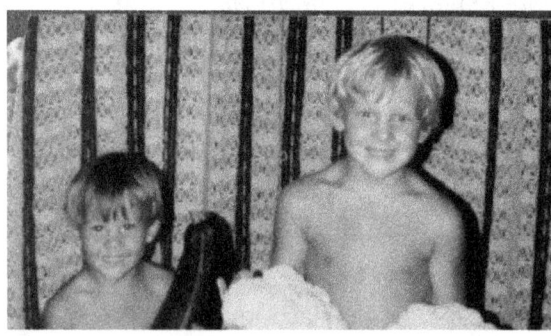

My brother and I were strong. He, much more so than I. He got the genes for size. I was the runt. He would often set up arm wrestling competitions for me with his friends, who were three or four years my elder. It was hilarious to him, watching his little freshman brother, take down seniors, to see their frustration and humiliation.

We were raised for strength…not health. I did okay as a college freshman, due to the fact that I attended a small private college that lacked some modern amenities, such as elevators. Seriously. And I lived on the fourth floor of the 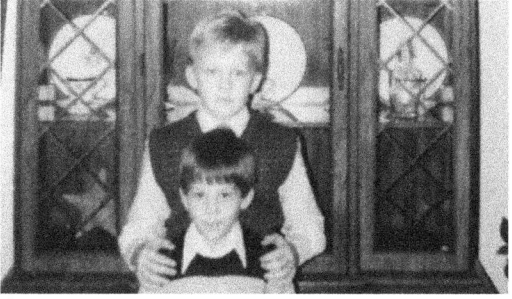 dorms. Also, the extra expense of attending a private college came with the perks of 3 homemade meals a day. St. Catharine's College sat on a three-hundred acre working farm that supplied the school fresh food for its staff and students. To make money I got a job, you guessed it, on a local farm. I was in the best shape of my life.

My second year of college was a drastic shift. I transferred to Eastern Kentucky University where there was no lack of modern amenities. I was now in the city. I grew accustom to eating in the food court with my friends, riding elevators, and scheduling my classes for more opportunity for sleep. I never had thought about the fact that the past was no predictor of the future and the joys of being fit could change. My sedentary lifestyle and increase in bad food choices began to create unappreciated changes in my body. For the next few years my weight went in one direction. Up. My health also went in one direction. Down.

Within the next three years I had met and married the woman of my dreams. I had met Mandy in college, while attending a Bible study in our campus ministry. We shared a love for the Lord and ministry and could see how He might use us to serve Him as husband and wife. We married the fall of 2001. I had been working in civil engineering while praying, to seek the Lord's direction for ministry opportunity. I had surrendered to a call on my life at the age of 18 to ministry and knew one day I would enter the pulpit to serve a church as pastor. I had given myself to every opportunity to serve, where I felt God had led me. I'd served as youth minister to a couple different churches; acted as a supply to preach in absence of pastors when called upon. Mandy and I were living a very good life as a newlywed couple.

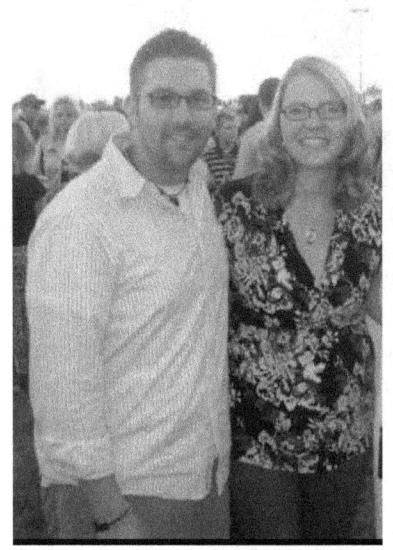

That December was unseasonably cold. Mandy and I were living in a partially furnished apartment that we had rented in Richmond, KY, home of our alma mater. We were still saving to buy more furniture and figuring out what this whole married thing was all about. I was dreading the alarm clock that morning, knowing that I would be working outside all that day in the cold. The phone call that I received proved to be more dreaded than any alarm clock. At 5am I got a call from my mother, frantic and inconsolable. Nearly a hundred miles away, my parents and brother still lived on my childhood farm. My brother Dustin, twenty-four, was still trying to find his way into adulthood, discerning a career path and hopeful future with his girlfriend at the time. The morning of December 19th, 2001, while on his way to work, he hit a spot of "black" ice. His truck slid one way, then the next. In a panic to control the vehicle he inadvertently overcorrected, sending the truck flipping and rolling through the air. Because he wasn't wearing his seat belt, he was ejected from the truck, landing some 40 feet away on the other side of the road from where the truck came to rest. He was air lifted from the scene to the University of Cincinnati Hospital with traumatic head and brain injury.

I hung up the phone, woke Mandy, and in a frenzy, departed at breakneck speeds to make it to the hospital. I was unaware of the extent of damage. I didn't know if he would be alive when I got there. I didn't know anything. Mandy prayed the entire way, both for my brother's life and for our safety as we weaved in and out of traffic, dismissing the speed limit.

When we arrived at the hospital, we met our family still waiting in the triage to hear some news of his condition. We cried and we prayed. We were told his chances of living another 24 hours were extremely slim, though, if he did, would mean a great deal about saving him. Eventually we were taken back to the Surgical Intensive Care unit where Dustin had been placed. I did not recognize him. His entire body was completely intact. Not even a scratch. But, his head, completely wrapped, was swollen to the size of a basketball. Upon being ejected from the truck, he had collided headfirst into a tree. As his brain swelled rapidly, in order to save his life, doctors had to cut away large portions of skull to relieve the expansive swelling. I had never seen a more gruesome and heartbreaking sight in all my life. I fell to my knees, weeping and praying.

Dustin was three years older than me and it had always been just the two of us. After my parents had me, I guess they decided that was all they could handle! He and I grew up sharing a bedroom and fighting constantly. At times you might have thought we even hated each other. That's what brothers do, I guess. As we grew and matured, we matured in our love and respect for one another. We weren't just brothers; we were best friends. We shared the same friends, hung out in the same places, attended concerts together. Just a few months earlier, Dustin was standing at my side as my best man in my wedding.

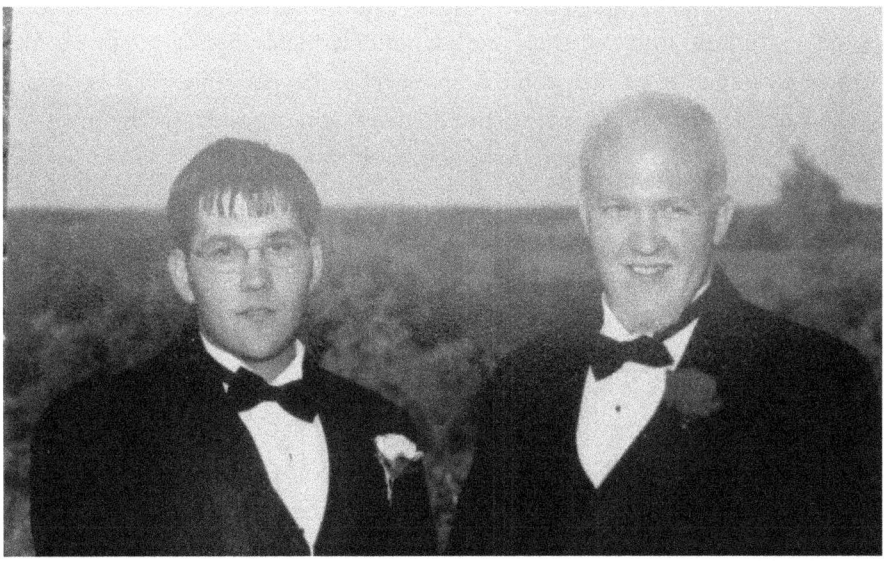

The moment he died was the most crushing blow I had ever received. I don't know if it was said aloud or just in my head, as I screamed to him, "Please don't leave me! I love you, Dustin! Please don't leave me! Oh God!" A feeling rushed over me that I had never felt, and one that I would not feel again for years to come. My hands began to tingle like cold stabbings from a thousand daggers. My breathing went shallow and rapid. Knees weakened, I slid down the wall. I felt like vomiting. I was in a panic.

After the funeral my parents and I with Mandy, sat in their living room staring at un-opened Christmas presents, some marked "TO: Dustin". One by one we opened them and cried. My mother took the gift from his boxes and gathered receipts for their return. My family would never be the same. My parents lost their firstborn child. I lost my leader and best friend. Our faith was shattered as we reeled in confusion and anger over unanswered prayers. Never before had we ever endured such a trial as this one.

I thought I was doing everyone a favor. My parents were so distraught by Dustin's death and I knew someone had to be strong for them. I voted for yours truly. I lay aside my grief and constantly reminded myself, my parents, and his friends that He was in a better place. I knew He was with Jesus, and God did heal him, ultimately. I consoled myself with those facts. I moved Mandy and myself home to be close to my parents and help to mend all our broken hearts. I cried in the shower where no one could hear me. At night I would venture off into the living room where I would bury my face in a throw pillow and wail in anguish. I would find myself alone, standing in his bedroom or the garage where he spent most of his time working and building projects. I would simply stand in silence, wrapped in hidden grief.

My dad taught me to be strong. I saw strength in him throughout my upbringing. He exemplified the highest pain tolerance of anyone I'd ever known. Now it was my turn to give back. I took all of my mourning and all of my anguish and I buried it deep. I mean deep, deep beneath everything in me. I focused on the things before me. A new wife, a new place to live, and soon, a new career.

Dustin died February 3rd, 2002. Just months after my marriage to Mandy. Following his death, I focused on what I was supposed to be doing in this life. Ministry. I simply reminded myself of the words of Jesus to "let the dead bury their dead. But you follow me." I misunderstood the meaning of what He said.

Just five months later Mandy and I moved again. This time would bring about an even greater change to our lives. We accepted the call of a nearly 200-year-old little church that sat along the Ohio River in a one-horse town known as Rabbit Hash. The church was a small country church that has seen very little change since the days its founding members dug and kiln fired earth to make bricks in which they built the church. I was happy and honored to finally have my chance at entering the ministry full-time. I would soon discover how undulating those feelings would be.

They were a loving church. As I look back, I pity them for having to put up with me for the time I spent as their pastor. Though I did my best, I was certainly a rookie preacher with a bit of a chip on my shoulder. Still carrying grief buried with me, the tendency to stress was amplified. I often felt like Bruce Banner, the human counterpart to the Incredible Hulk; constantly working to keep the monster within at bay. I would faithfully teach Sunday morning Bible classes for our youth, preach two sermons on Sunday, lead a mid-week Bible study, stay active making visits to shut-ins and nursing homes and hospital patients. At night I would collapse into my bed with a bottle of Pepto-Bismol on my nightstand and rolls of Tums antacids.

The demanding schedule of a pastor does not lend itself to a healthy lifestyle. Constantly on the road, or in between responsibilities I found myself still eating convenient processed junk. My weight, ever climbing, had peaked at 200 pound plus. My energy levels were depleted, my emotional hygiene suffering, and the news of a baby on the way…it was high time I did something.

Mandy and I decided to join a gym. Even though we made very little money, hardly enough to survive on, we felt this was a worthy investment. Every morning at 5am we made our way to a new 'globo' gym about 20 minutes away. There, we were greeted by a muscle bound, retired competition bodybuilder named Franco. Not Franco Columbo. This Franco was working on commission and super excited to sign us up. He quickly took us through some basic circuit weight moves and took a rough measurement of our body fat. I needed work. I hadn't lifted or been active since college.

We also heard about a new diet that everyone seemed to be talking about. The Adkins Diet was all the rage. Dr. Adkins and his team had devised an eating plan that seemed to just melt fat right off a person. The catch? Extremely low carb. This didn't translate with my brain; a brain that had been carb loaded and carb addicted since childhood. My food pyramid at this time consisted of pizza (foundationally of course), pasta, tortilla chips, and French fries. Nevertheless, I was desperate. We printed out some recipes, went grocery shopping, and got to work. Morning breakfasts were a delight. Eggs, bacon, and lots of Jimmy Dean Country Sausage! Yum! Lunch was similar. At dinner we tried our hand at some of these "less than traditional" dishes. We could not get a handle on the spaghetti squash spaghetti. We found crustless pizza. Meh, that's not as good as my regular pizza, but let's give it a go.

Weight began to drop. Dr. Adkin's diet seemed to be my answer. Working out regularly had seemed to help with energy. Still, none of that seemed to be helping my heart. I continued to grow weary and frustrated. Yes, I thought I was doing well physically, but I wasn't. I had no plan when going to the gym. I had no idea what I was doing. My diet was low carb, but it was far from healthy. I maintained highly oxidized stress, inflammation, and little to no recovery. Fat loss does not equate to good health. The "patches" that I tried did not last. It's easy to blame finances on the lack of gym involvement. Nutritionally, well that failure was simply a lack of education. Now, I'm not knocking Dr. Adkins or his diet approach. I actually respect it greatly. But, without any understanding of nutrition and nutritional value, I only ended up eating a high protein diet full of junk protein and rancid, inflammatory fats and oils. What I had intended to be my catalyst to healing and better health only exasperated the issues.

We spent three years serving the people at that little country church and Rabbit Hash. With our first newborn son in our lives, we felt an overwhelming relief to accept a call to a church closer to home. Grandparents are a wonderful thing to have around! We moved back to my hometown, near my parents, where I would accept the position of associate pastor. Jackpot! I felt like this was God smiling down upon us. We had endured so many hardships for the past several years, and now we get some relief. The church provided a decent salary, a parsonage to live in, and as the associate pastor I didn't have to carry the load of leadership, not the target on my back.

Little did I know, before my arrival, there was internal conflict, building pressure of seismic proportions. The deacons were unhappy with the current pastor, who, was not only my boss but my friend. Within a few months of my tenure, and hoping for some relief, there was a call for the pastor to resign or be fired.

The pastor resigned. The deacons were satisfied with their actions, the pastor and his wife forever injured by them. As I stood in the middle of this explosion and attempting to discern a clear path, I was uncertain. I had believed with all my heart that God called me to this church. At this point, though, I wasn't sure they even needed my position. The congregation had dwindled. To pay an associate pastor seemed unnecessary and the deacons agreed. Instead they asked me to stay and continue on as their pastor. Mandy and I prayed about this long and hard. It only seemed right to us to stay and help lead the church to a healthy place and considering the fact that God hadn't opened any other doors for us, we accepted.

Being in a bigger church and a bigger community didn't make my life better, it made it busier. The business and activity kept me occupied. Mandy was now pregnant with our second son and I was growing as a community leader. We bolstered our church growth and expanded ministries. I was able to hire a worship leader and break ground on a multi-purpose building that would double the size of our current structure. Baptisms were up. Way up. We were helping the church transition and develop as a healthy, community-oriented church.

I set out to create what would be the community's first and only drug rehabilitation ministry. In December of 2006 I started Reach of Northern Kentucky. Better known as 'Reach', we hosted weekly outpatient support meetings, low cost drug testing, and gave 100% scholarships for those who wanted and needed in-patient care.

Next, I helped to start a new community food and clothing pantry that would serve the entire community in giving away free food, clothing, and toiletries to any and all who were in need. Meeting the Needs Ministry, as well as REACH are still active today.

After that, I helped to launch Hope's Hands, a community collaborative that assisted families and youth by bringing together all our local resources responsible for serving them.

All the while, receiving a Bachelor of Theology degree from seminary. Needless to say, I stayed busy. That business felt great. It successfully took my mind off my demons…or so I thought.

The body has a funny way of telling you something is wrong. By 2007-2008 I had reached my fat gain pinnacle. I weighed in at 226 pounds, a full 60 pounds more than my high school graduating weight. My diet was not any better. Honestly, it was worse. Fast food giant hamburger value meals and frozen pizzas were my staple diet. Zero exercise.

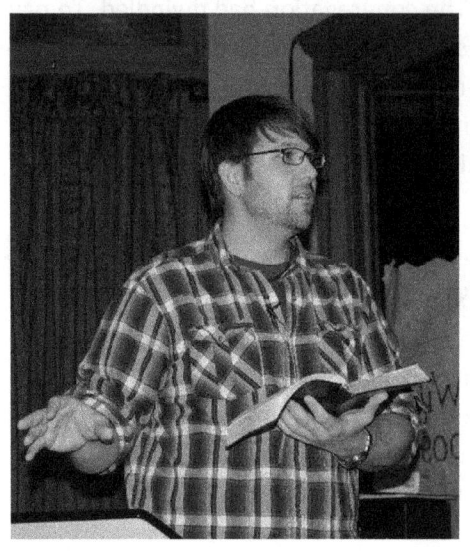

One night on a camping a trip with our church youth group, my body decided to tell me something was wrong. While the kids slept peacefully in their tents circled around a dying campfire, I was lying inside a cozy RV camper with my youth leaders, thinking I was dying! Out of nowhere, and in the middle of the night I turned from Dr. Jekyll to Mr. Hyde. I began to feel an irritating itch on the back of my neck. Soon it spread to my waistband, then by groin, and then everywhere. I was covered in hives. Then, following this outbreak, my stomach began to cramp and become extremely nauseated. Then, my hands began to constrict and contort as if I were being electrocuted. I couldn't open my fingers and control my reflexes. My breathing began to grow shallow and rapid "What is happening to me!", I thought. After a while, things settled down and I did not need medical treatment. I made it through the night.

My assumption was that I must have encountered some allergen. My body simply, rejected it and had an allergic reaction. I blamed in on the probability of a reaction to cedar trees or campfire smoke. I don't know...it sounded plausible.

Not long after that episode, I found myself in the bathroom at home at 3 am. Every symptom was back, except worsened. Everything I mentioned that happened before was happening again, but with a vengeance. This time around I endured vomiting and diarrhea simultaneously. My hands again contorted, burned. I ran cold water over my hands that now felt like they were being dipped in acid. The event came and went, like before. Mysterious. There were no cedar trees or campfire. I had done nothing out of the norm that day. "Am I going crazy?" I thought. I kept quiet and didn't tell anyone other than Mandy.

These episodes persisted and worsened over the months.

In the summer of 2008, God had developed my heart and helped me to discover my knack for entrepreneurial leadership. I enjoy creating new ministries, organizations, and movements. I also had an extraordinary desire to see people come to know Jesus. I was frustrated at the limitations to this goal that we, as the church, had self-imposed through traditions. While I loved my church and the people, I could not sleep at night thinking of ways we could better reach our communities for Christ. I had never considered church planting. It was never something that was really talked about. In my head, that was a movement long ago that was responsible for starting all our current churches. Now, it is our responsibility to 'grow' these churches. Yes, I was so naive! God began to show me the success rates of new churches verses the growth of older, established churches. He often moves by using frustration. He causes me to be unsettled with where I am currently, then gives me a vision of where I need to go. Then, He waits for me to step out.

That October I stepped out. I resigned from a healthy church that paid a great salary to begin the work of starting a church, receiving no salary. I walked away from my job and home. I needed to find employment and housing for my wife and two babies, quick!

My parents raised me with specific values and ethics. Whether they did it by voicing them through their teaching, or by exemplifying them through their actions, they were no less engrained in me. The two that stand out? Hard work and honesty. These are essential. They are non-negotiable. They are two of my essential core values.

It is those values that I used to start Epoch Fellowship Church. (Epoch that sounds like 'epic'). Mandy and I listened to our mentors, followed our denominational guides, and went to work. I had never planted a church before. What does it take to build a church from the ground up? Oh, and work two other jobs, raise two toddlers, be a husband, and be in bad health? Hard work and honesty? Right?

We developed a core team of interested co-laborers of about 25 who would serve as our starter congregation, our set-up and break-down crew, as well as our babysitters. The local high school gave us the use of their two-hundred and fifty seat, state of the art auditorium to use for our Sunday night services, as well as our Tuesday youth meetings. Every Sunday afternoon, we would load up all our sound equipment and decorations form storage, drive to the school where we would begin set up. Afterwards, we would break it all back down and take it back to storage. It was hard work, but we were thankful to have such a nice facility that lent itself to potential growth.

Later we found, what had actually been a church, left vacant and abandoned, located on a piece of developmental property. We were able to secure it within a week of our departure from the school. We signed a rent to buy agreement, securing a future. The building, once owned by a church, had been left vacant for several years. Structurally it was sound, but we needed to do quite a bit of updating. We spent the next two months renovating. Walls were painted, lights hung, youth and nursery rooms assembled, and lots and lots of TLC. And money. We spent lots of money to get this place ready for worship. We installed all new audio equipment, bought furniture, and made repairs. By the time we were done, we had a very nice place to finally call our own.

We had spent two months renovating our new place. Another two months spent using it to grow our congregation. We had been asked to help out on a Sunday afternoon in our community to park, to volunteer with a family event taking place. There were games, crafts, food, and a great band…ours. Our church had a great day. That night was even better. The house was packed. You could just sense the excitement and joy in the air. Two months into our new location and we were finally hitting our stride. I was working as a substitute teacher at the time to help meet our financial needs. The following morning from our Sunday evening service, I was up getting ready for work when my phone rang. It was one of our members who also worked at the school. As I answered the phone, I heard the following, "Brother Trent, the church is on fire! It's burning!"

I hurried to the site to find firefighters working the fire, trying to get it contained. The building, built in the eighties was a metal sided building; great for strength, though, a nightmare in case of fire. I immediately instructed my executive pastor to contact the insurance company and notify them of our loss in hopes of rebuilding eventually. That idea burned down as well. Fine print is a son of a gun. Yes, we were insured. However, our belongings were only insured if they were on the property of our mother or sponsoring church, which obviously they were not. We didn't own the building. As a matter of fact, we were supposed to. Our closing date on our purchase was overshot by about three days because the team of developers which owned the building had dragged their feet. Re-building, then, would be up to them. They decided that it would not be in their best interest to build, as the building itself was not worth anything to them. The land however was their investment, and without the building, it made the value of the land more. We could still purchase the land, as they offered, only now for a much heftier price than before. Bigger price tag, no building

We had come so far. How could this have happened? What would we do? Well, in my mind there was only one answer. Persevere. I was not raised to be a quitter. We would just put in the work and do what we needed to do. I mean, God would only expect nothing short of excellence, right?

We spent the next year borrowing space in a local church, who had graciously donated to us on Sunday evenings. As we began the work of a new church, much of the community saw it as a threat. To my surprise and disappointment. I hadn't considered the fact that there had not been a church planted in this community within any of the current living generation's lifetime. It was a totally alien idea. Sure, new churches had been started, but by the result of some church split. When we decided to start a totally new work, we were seen as an insult. Almost as to say, "You all are wrong, or not working, and we are here to do it right and better." Many of my pastor friends who I had for years grown to love and trust as friends, turned on me. Some stopped talking to me and avoided me. Others took up talking about me. When our building burned it was said that God burned us down. And as a warning to other churches, not to have anything to do with us, or God would burn them down as well.

I became the subject of small-town gossip. My name was whispered around town and on-line. I was called a cult leader and my church was called a cult. Rumors began to spread, accusing me of extra-marital affairs and all sorts of evil, nasty things. One rumor in particular was that I had stolen a person's dog! I endured, and I put on a brave face, but these attacks and shunnings were becoming more than I could withstand. I never fought back or retaliated. I hid the hurt and went on.

After a year of borrowing space, we were finally able to acquire our own again. We were thrilled. The location was perfect. We found a store front building located right in the middle of downtown. It had been used to house a communications business and was in no way ready to house a church. I did what I did best. I rolled up my sleeves and went to work renovating. Mandy says that she lost her husband during those days. She is right. I worked around the clock. During the day I worked two jobs and pastored our church. At night I worked as a remodeler. I spent every waking hour I could to get this church back online once again. Would God expect anything less?

I was so hurt by the community gossip that I kept myself away from public as much as possible. I would dart in and out of buildings, avoid stores, and plan my routes in order to steer clear from the looks and jeers. My perceptions grew to absurdity. It felt like everyone hated me, though, I know in reality they didn't. To build this church and to be successful in it, was almost a "righteous" way of defeating my enemies. It was vain glory.

We completed the building, making it into a super cool coffee shop that we named The Wild Goose Café, based on the name used by ancient Celtic Christians' term for the Holy Spirit. We wanted to be active in the community, though I led from behind the scenes, and radically change the culture of our community to know and see the power of God. We opened as a café to serve the community during the week and our church used it for worship services on the weekends and mid-week. It was a novel approach to ministry, and I was proud of it. I had never managed a café before, but we were looking to utilize our resources and my creative entrepreneurship to capitalize on Kingdom growth. Though now, it meant more work. But isn't that what God would want?

I had started this church in October of 2008. God blessed our efforts and honored His vision and the church grew and was healthy. Its pastor wasn't. We had suffered so may fatal setbacks and overcame them. We dealt with serious external attacks and ignored them. By year three, I was done.

They say there are signs that help predict destructive geographical phenomenon. Earthquakes, tsunamis, volcanic eruptions; though nearly impossible to predict, there are early warning signs that give off indications that something is about to break loose. Time, pressure, and a trigger. That's all it takes.

Ten years earlier I dealt with the most devastating event in my life with the loss of my brother. At the time, I sequestered my grieving in an attempt to be strong and do what needed to be done for others. I was satisfied that I done a good job at this. Over the years I thought less and less of my brother. I convinced myself that I had simply healed and moved on.

Over the course of those previous ten years I lived in a state of chronic stress and an activated, over run parasympathetic nervous system. My adrenal glands, which are responsible for regulating stress hormones such as adrenaline and cortisol, were taxed. I suffered adrenal fatigue. Symptoms often revealed themselves with abdominal weight gain, fatigue, moodiness, and low libido. After one routine examination, one of my care providers actually said to me, "you love what you do, but what you do is killing you. You have forgotten how to relax and play." He was right. The stress, like my grief was suppressed and internalized. By looking on the outside, you would not have guessed what was going on in my body.

By holding onto the chronic stress, I put pressure on my adrenals, which caused numerous problems. On top of that, my lumbar spine did two things. It twisted at the L4-L5 and kinked, creating a bout of scoliosis and constant pain. The pain persisted to the point that I struggled getting in and out of the car. Sleep was hindered as well. At times the pain would take my breath away. Time had built up. Pressure had peaked. I began to have panic attacks. I had only ever had one in my life, ten years earlier standing in a SICU hospital ward. Even then I didn't know what it was. Out of nowhere, and for no known reason, my heart would begin to race, my breathing would grow rapid and shallow, and my hands would go numb.

Then the trigger.

Mandy and the boys, along with two friends of ours, decided to take a vacation to Hilton Head, South Carolina. There, my mother-in-law owned a beautiful condo in a lush resort with its own private beach. Simply paradise. We booked the week, headed down, and enjoyed several glorious days in the sun, on a private beach and lots of Putt-Putt golf. The weather was perfect and everyday was exactly what we needed. They say there is a calm before the storm. Just before the great calamity is a sense of peace or stillness. Near the end of the week, we sat exhausted back at the condo. Deciding to stay in for the night we voted on junk food and a movie. I grabbed the keys, jumped in the car and headed off to the nearby grocery store. With ice cream, pizza, and a movie in tow, I jumped back in the car and sat there for just a moment. Out of nowhere I had a glimmering thought of my brother. It surprised me. I hadn't been talking about him. Nothing that I saw or did reminded me of him. It was just as if a tiny pinhole had broken the surface of a barrier that had been holding back a lake of emotions of ten years. I began to cry.

I sat in the car for what seemed like hours, though maybe a couple minutes in reality. The tears would not stop. I wasn't even sure where they were coming from. I managed to put my finger in the pinhole long enough to head back to the condo. No one was the wiser. We continued with the night, and after the movie as everyone was cleaning up from the sprawl of gluttonous junk food, I made my way out to the balcony. I stood, staring off into the distance. Mandy approached me from behind and placed her hand on my back. I busted. Tears once again began to flow. I was shocked and embarrassed. Mandy stood in shock as well, having no idea why I was upset. I had no idea why I was upset. The tears continued. Again, I managed to gain my composure and plug the hole. "What is going on?", I thought.

After we had arrived back home in Kentucky, I thought perhaps I had experienced a couple little, odd incidents while on vacation. I was wrong. The dam busted. What had been pent up inside of me for ten years decided that that was long enough. This time there was no managing it or holding it back. I had become inconsolable. Every detail of grief that I thought I had buried with my brother emerged with a vengeance. My heart, completely broken, and my emotions shattered, I became virtually non-functioning. I had no idea how to deal with these emotions, let alone explain them. I lashed out at close friends, and alienated others. I became a social nightmare. The only time that I was able to remotely function was when I was in "pastoring" mode. Still able to preach, I adopted the mindset of "fake it 'til you make it." I couldn't let all of this dampen what I was doing for God. I needed to present to Him a wonderful church. I needed to perform at a high level for Him. I needed Him to be proud of me. That is what He would want, right?

Feeling the need to perform, all the while my emotional lake was being drained, my body begin to turn on itself. The peculiar attacks of hives, nausea, vomiting, etcetera, worsened. I started to research my symptoms intensely. Little made sense. Finally, I stumbled upon a rare genetic disorder. It fit perfectly. I made an appointment with my family physician and we went over my case. It seemed to fit an auto-immune disorder known as Hereditary Angioedema. According to the Genetic and Rare Disease Information Center, Hereditary Angioedema is a "disease characterized by recurrent episodes (also called attacks) of severe swelling of the skin and mucous membranes. The age at which attacks begin varies, but most people have their first one in childhood or adolescence. The frequency of attacks usually increases after puberty.

Attacks most often affect 3 parts of the body:

- Skin - the most common sites are the face (such as the lips and eyes), hands, arms, legs, genitals, and buttocks. Skin swelling can cause pain, dysfunction, and disfigurement.

- Gastrointestinal tract - the stomach, intestines, bladder, and/or urethra may be involved. This may cause symptoms such as nausea, vomiting, diarrhea, and abdominal pain.

- Upper airway (such as the larynx and tongue) - this can cause upper airway obstruction and may be life-threatening. The majority of attacks affecting the airway resolve before complete airway obstruction.

Attacks may involve one area of the body at a time, or they may involve a combination of areas. They always go away on their own but last from 2 to 4 days. While people with HAE have reported various triggers of attacks, emotional stress, and physical stress are the most commonly reported triggers." [1]

After further testing I was diagnosed with type 3 Hereditary Angioedema. In short (and without all the "sciency" stuff) I developed a genetic mutation in my F12 gene, which, once activated sends misinformed information to my body that causes it to attack itself. Specifically promoting inflammation by increasing the permeability of blood vessel walls, allowing more fluids to leak into body tissues. This leakage causes the swelling that accompanies inflammation. The stomach pain, nausea, and gastric distress is from blood rushing into my intestines, causing severe swelling of the intestinal walls. As if the prognosis wasn't bad enough, I received even worse news. There's no cure. The disease can be mitigated with frozen plasma transfusions that have a specific gene type but, there was no such plasma available in Kentucky. My only hope was an epinephrine pen. In the event that during an attack my airway swelled shut, I was instructed to inject myself with a dose of epinephrine to relieve the attack and 'hopefully' save my life. At the time HEA boasted a thirty percent fatality rate.

I dealt with regular attacks, which increased in pain and duration. The more attacks I had the more depressed I become. It was a vicious cycle. I had a disease that was triggered by emotional stress that caused more emotional stress. As soon as a new attack begin, I wondered if this would be the one that would kill me. The attacks grew so excruciatingly painful, that while I was having them, I literally prayed to God that it would.

I lost any and all foreseeable future of hope. My depression deepened as I became isolated and withdrawn. At night, to avoid my family after work, I would fill a bathtub with hot water and soak for hours. In those moments of despair, I remember sliding my body down where my face would be at water level and just think to myself, "just one large breath of water…just fill your lungs, and die." There were days I would be driving to work, and I would hold the accelerator down until reaching speeds of close to 100. Then I would think, "Just a quick whip of the steering wheel. It'll all be over in a second." My mind drifted into the deepest, darkest recesses of depression and anguish I had ever known. I stopped looking at people and only looked through them. My world had no color, only black.

I kept journal entries of thoughts and musings and as I drifted into this soul eating despair, it was reflected in my writing.

JULY 2, 2011

I'LL KILL MYSELF FOR WHAT I LOVE. I'M JUST NOT SURE I'LL RESURRECT AFTERWARDS.

NOVEMBER 15, 2011
THIS DAY WILL END NEXT WEEK.
Sleepless
Nauseous
Restless

NOVEMBER 21, 2011

Dear Sleep,

I miss you. We used to be so good together. Remember when I'd just fall into you? Where did you go? Any more I feel like I spend half the night chasing you. To little avail. Are my thoughts keeping you away? There's so many. It'd be rude to tell them all to be quiet. I've been doubling up on your aids. Am I going to have to triple up? I can't get enough of you. I'd like to meet you again. Try not to stay away anymore.

Yours Truly

DECEMBER 3, 2011

DISTANT & DISCONNECTED

DECEMBER 6, 2011

BAD DIET + LACK OF SLEEP+ EMOTIONAL STRESS = DEPLETED IMMUNE SYSTEM

Which is why I have a low-grade fever, headache, aches, pains and exhaustion. I need to sleep about 3 solid days.

DECEMBER 28, 2011

CONFESSION IS GOOD FOR THE SOUL

It's no secret that due to my high stress lifestyle that I've incurred a bit of the reactions to some of that stress. My body has taken its toll, among other things. I tend to take things personally or hold on to things and dwell on them until havoc be wreaked on me. Ironically enough the greatest stress has come largely due to relationships and where my life touches other people's lives. It's ironic because I've been termed 'relationally autistic' as a dear sentiment. Yet being acutely gifted in sociology hasn't voided the stress that 'social' puts on me. And so here of late I've been praying a very seemingly bad prayer though harboring what I hope is good intentions. "Lord, help me to care less." On the surface that seems bad. We should care. But I'm afraid I may care too much for the wrong things. The things that damage my adrenal glands. I truly do care greatly for mortal man and his eternal destiny. Let that be my focus. Perhaps a broader brush stroke. And thus, I have felt, whether by divinity or personal sanity, the growth of a certain apathy in my heart. It could be a letting go period. Perhaps a giving in or giving up. I'm not quite sure. But one thing is for sure. There are certain days when caring less about the things that cause the stress is a relief in and of itself.

FEBRUARY 16, 2012

I'M GOING TO FREE FALL OUT INTO NOTHING.

I'm going to leave this world for a while.

- Tom Petty

At this point, darkness had enveloped me like a blanket. I could not hear God. I could not feel Him. I cried out, no avail. My mind was wrecked by depression. My body was wrecked by stress and disease. One fateful night as I lay in bed, I was awoken by a slight itch around my waistband. Following was another on the back of my head. I knew what was coming. In a matter of minutes my entire body was covered in burning, itching hives. My intestines filling with blood, I ran to the bathroom ready for vomiting and/or diarrhea. Mandy had developed a system by this point. She had the epi-pen ready just in case. "Here, take these." She handed me two Benadryl tablets. My body was on fire. My breathing starting to shallow. Mandy began to fill a bathtub with cold water, ready to plunge me in in hopes of relieving the symptoms. I stepped into the water. Knives slicing through my skin as the water touched the burning hives. I soaked and shivered, praying for relief. "I cannot do this anymore." I whimpered. And I couldn't. I began to climb out of the tub with little to no strength. Then I collapsed. When Mandy turned the corner, there, she found me lying, shivering on a cold bathroom floor, weeping uncontrollably. Without my heart ever stopping, and for all intents and purposes... I died. That night, I died a death much worse than physically death.

The accumulative years of emotional stress and unattended grief, unhealthy eating habits, lack of exercise, and dealing with a genetic disease left me a near ruined human being. It is a sheer miracle that it didn't ruin my marriage and ministry. Only by the grace of God. Now, you may be asking the question, "What does all this have to do with food?" By now, this all seems like a book about emotional health. Well, it is. Or, you may, by now, see it as a book on spiritual health and theology. Yes, it is that as well. You might be struggling to see how it could be a book about nutrition, diet, and physical health.

Holistic health is all of those things. My struggles weren't simply psychological issues. Nor were they only physical issues. Everything was intertwined. Every issue touched an area of my being; physical, emotional, and spiritual. And every issue was caused by every area of my being. My road to recovery was a long one. It was complex and touched many levels of healing. I had wonderful, godly people walk with me and support me. But, the road to recovery must start with taking the first step. This is the most important step. My goal in recovery, and finding my way again, was to re-discover myself and my Creator. I desired to heal from my brother's tragic death. That was needed. I had to find relief to my low back issues and adrenal depletion. I desperately needed to lose the extra sixty pounds of fat I was carrying. But, more than anything, I needed to discover who I was in Christ, and heal my relationship with God. Without that, none of my other needs or desires would ever have the possibility of seeing recovery.

My first step to recovery was the most essential and fundamental step. And it started with food. Where most people will advocate alternative healing practices first, such as counselling, drugs, and self-help books, (and all those things have their place), I am going to show you that food can and will be your road to recovery spiritually, physically, and emotionally. Food. It's the first innate desire that we longed for as we entered this world as babies. Could it hold the key to preventing stories like mine? Could it hold the key to recovering optimal holistic health? I believe it does.

You will begin to see how the food that you eat will reflect health in all areas of your life, either working for you or against you. You will also discover why food and the act of eating was intended in the first place. How food is meant to connect you to your Creator, and yet when mistreated, it often does the opposite. Shattered, broken, depressed, and in full-time ministry. This was my life at one point. How did I get here?

It is a statement not to be understated, or underestimated…

"You are what you eat."

Chapter 2

The Beginning Plate
(Food's Role in Establishing a Relationship With God And His People)

"Owners of dogs will have noticed that, if you provide them with food and water and shelter and affection, they will think you are god. Whereas owners of cats are compelled to realize that, if you provide them with food and water and shelter and affection, they draw the conclusion that they are gods."

— Christopher Hitchens, *The Portable Atheist: Essential Readings for the Nonbeliever*

As odd as it may seem to quote an atheist, Hitchens actually brings about a profound point that Christians need to ask and consider. Did God establish food and diet so that we may know His greatness, or that we may assume our own? Think about it...why did God even create the idea and function of eating? Why not just create biological beings to be like Superman who gets his energy and strength from the Sun? When creating all things, when it comes to the engineering of biology, an infinite, all powerful Creator could have done it any way He wanted. It would certainly be easier for us, if when we are tired or hungry, to simply go out for a little sunbathing action and allow photosynthesis or solar charging to satiate us instead of having to worry about what our next meal would be or from where it would come. Whoa! Hold on! There it is. There's the point. Jesus makes it very clear to us.

"This is why I tell you: Don't worry about your life, what you will eat or what you will drink; or about your body, what you will wear. Isn't life more than food and the body more than clothing? Look at the birds of the sky: They don't sow or reap or gather into barns, yet your heavenly Father feeds them. Aren't you worth more than they?"
Matthew 6:25, 26

Or how about when asked by His disciples how to pray and He answers,

"Therefore, you should pray like this: 'Our Father in heaven, your name be honored as holy. Your kingdom come. Your will be done on earth as it is in heaven. Give us today our daily bread.'"
Matthew 6:9-11

Just like a newborn baby, who is completely dependent upon their mother to feed them, we are taught to rely and trust on God for our every meal! Every meal enjoyed by a newborn baby suckling its mother's milk points to an intimate but silent dialogue with the child saying, "Mom, you are faithful to me." and the mother replying, "You are worthy of my faithfulness." Every meal of our life is a teaching moment where God shows us His faithfulness to provide what is necessary in our lives as well as the level of value He puts on us. Every meal is God's way of showing off His power, not yours. It shows us a daily dependency on God to supply our every need, even the most basic. And if lived out in such a way, we would be freed up enough from worrying about ourselves to be able to spend that time on Him, spending that time with Him. So, let's go back to the beginning to see the establishment of God's relationship with mankind through food and diet.

"Then God said, 'Let us make man in Our image, according to Our likeness. They will rule the fish of the sea, the birds of the sky, the livestock, the whole earth, and the creatures that crawl on the earth.' So God created man in his own image; he created him in the image of God; he created them male and female. God blessed them, and God said to them, 'Be fruitful, multiply, fill the earth, and subdue it. Rule the fish of the sea, the birds of the sky, and every creature that crawls on the earth.' God also said, 'Look, I have given you every seed-bearing plant on the surface of the entire earth and every tree whose fruit contains seed. This will be food for you, for all the wildlife of the earth, for every bird of the sky, and for every creature that crawls on the earth—everything having the breath of life in it—I have given every green plant for food.'"
Genesis 1:26-30

Imagine if you will how all this plays out. God is at work creating our world and everything in it. Upon creating the first man, Adam and his wife Eve, He blesses them with authority of the responsibility of stewardship of His creation and then He gives them a gift: food. He could have offered them anything under the sun. As the crowning achievement of his creation, He could have gifted them with anything: tools, technology, powers, or for that matter, clothing! But no, He gifts them with an endless supply of food that they will never have to work for. This food was the first gift, a gift meant to teach them that He desired constant fellowship and total dependence. What a joy to never have to worry about cooking! They would never have to worry about where they would eat, how they would eat, what they would eat, or even what was in their food. It was all for them, and all perfect! What a life. Aside from the marriage relationship that God gave as a holy institution to Adam and Eve, food was the greatest and most sacred gift given to them. It was given that they would know their worth, and His faithfulness.

"The Lord God planted a garden in Eden, in the east, and there he placed the man he had formed. The Lord God caused to grow out of the ground every tree pleasing in appearance and good for food, including the tree of life in the middle of the garden, as well as the tree of the knowledge of good and evil."
Genesis 2:8-9

"And the Lord God commanded the man, 'You are free to eat from any tree of the garden, but you must not eat from the tree of the knowledge of good and evil, for on the day you eat from it, you will certainly die.'"
Genesis 2:16-17

How important is food? As we have already seen, it is necessary for life. We've also seen how God chose to use it as a daily teaching on his love for us and his faithfulness to us. But notice too, how food is used as His first and only command to Adam. My son, who is just a young child but already a deep thinker, asked me just the other day, "If God knew Adam was going to sin, then why did He even make him?" What a wonderful question! I posed this question back to him, "Would you rather be able to choose to love me, or be forced to love me?" He immediately spoke up, "Choose to love you!" "Well, son, by God giving Adam this one commandment, He was giving Adam the ability to choose to love and obey Him or choose to disobey Him." That answer seemed to make sense to him. But why was God's one command- his one instruction to NOT do something revolve around a fruit tree? Was it poison and was God only looking after Adam's physical well-being? If we read on, we see in verse 6 of chapter 3, "The woman saw that the tree was good for food ..." No, this fruit was not poisonous or toxic. And maybe THAT was part of the point! It stands to reason that God would apply His one commandment surrounding the one thing in creation that could compete with man's love for him...food. Adam and Eve were human beings, with human appetites. They surely ate daily meals and grew accustom to trying new things and experiencing new tastes. Food was made attractive, and full of pleasure as a means to bless Adam and his wife. Food was a necessity AND a blessing. So, imagine how important food must have been for the very first and only restriction God implemented was to be a dietary restriction. This was sure to test man's love, loyalty, and ability to not sin. Why, he would surely have to be a most perfect and upright being if he could keep THIS command! It shouldn't surprise us, that humans have been failing at trying to keep a diet from the very beginning, so don't be too hard on yourself when you find yourself giving in.

Food was used by God to establish a love relationship with the first man. I believe that shows its importance. However, it didn't end there. Food was also used as a way to establish a relationship of distinction with His people, the Israelites. Just a quick survey through the Biblical books of the Levitical laws, you will notice that there are quite a few dietary laws. Laws of food such as the type of "clean or unclean" food, and how to kill and finish the accepted animals for food. God even used diet to make a distinction between those He called His and those He did not. We have to conclude that the entire idea of food and everything revolving around it is of massive importance to spiritual well-being and not just physiological functioning.

For the establishment of His people, the Jews received dietary laws and requirements that set them apart from the rest of the world. A food that it considered 'abiding' by these regulations is considered "Kosher". Often times, people have speculated that these laws had to do with God's attention to healthy eating. This is not so. For instance, God commands the Israelites not to eat certain meat such as camel and rabbit. [Of the "beasts of the earth" (which basically refers to land mammals with the exception of swarming rodents), you may eat any animal that has cloven hooves and chews its cud. Lev. 11:3; Deut. 14:6. Any land mammal that does not have both of these qualities is forbidden. The Old Testament specifies that the camel and the rabbit are not kosher because they lack one of these two qualifications. Cattle, sheep, goats, deer and bison are kosher. From a health standpoint, camel and rabbit meat is no less healthy or nutritional than cow or deer. Further requirements involve birds and fowl, fish, and even insects. Many of which are given absolutely no reason for their distinction. And the rules don't only apply to foods that are permitted to be eaten, but parts of certain animals, instructions for processing, and even using utensils. Here are some guidelines that are to be followed:

1. Certain animals may not be eaten at all. This restriction includes the flesh, organs, eggs and milk of the forbidden animals.
2. Of the animals that may be eaten, the birds and mammals must be killed in accordance with Jewish law.
3. All blood must be drained from meat and poultry or broiled out of it before it is eaten.
4. Certain parts of permitted animals may not be eaten.
5. Fruits and vegetables are permitted, but must be inspected for bugs (which cannot be eaten)
6. Meat (the flesh of birds and mammals) cannot be eaten with dairy. Fish, eggs, fruits, vegetables and grains can be eaten with either meat or dairy. (According to some views, fish may not be eaten with meat).
7. Utensils (including pots and pans and other cooking surfaces) that have come into contact with meat may not be used with dairy, and vice versa. Utensils that have come into contact with non-kosher food may not be used with kosher food. This applies only where the contact occurred while the food was hot.
8. Grape products made by non-Jews may not be eaten.
9. There are a few other rules that are not universal. [1]

Admittedly, there are many health reasons behind some of God's regulations. His instructions of processing an animal are so healthy and sanitary that kosher butchers and slaughterhouses have been exempted from many USDA regulations. The quick and immediate drainage of blood from an animal prevents certain hormones and toxins from collecting in the meat. A kosher butcher knows to trim off all of the visceral fat that lines the internal organs of an animal, while leaving the subcutaneous fat that is found directly under the skin. The early Jews may not have known what science has only recently discovered, that there is a big difference between these two types of fat, and that the non-permissible visceral fat is more toxic to the animal, (and the one consuming it).

However, we also know that there are no scientific or health related reasons known, not given, for many of these laws. Could it be more of a utilitarian reason? Sure, a camel would serve better as a beast of burden rather than a pig. But then, that rule certainly wouldn't apply to a rabbit.

The simplest explanation for why Jews follow the long list of kosher dietary laws found in Scripture, Because God said so. In his book "To Be a Jew," Rabbi Hayim Halevy Donin suggests that the dietary laws are designed as a call to holiness. The ability to distinguish between right and wrong, good and evil, pure and defiled, the sacred and the profane, is very important in Judaism. Imposing rules on what you can and cannot eat ingrains that kind of self-control, requiring us to learn to control even our most basic, primal instincts.

Kosher law was God's way of sanctifying, or setting apart, His people with a specific and unique identity. Without giving them reasons for many of His requirements, they were to choose whether or not they were simply going to trust, believe, and obey, or not. In this way, the everyday ordinary act of eating was nothing less than an extraordinary act of religious devotion to the One they would follow. To the Jew, the act of eating could not have been done without a constant reminder that he or she was in fact a Jew. Food created their identity in the Lord. To break the law of diet would be to abandon the law of God and disband their identity in Him. Daniel, while exiled to Babylon, was so resolute in his identity in the Lord, that he refused the King's meat and risked losing his life. How would you view food, if by the way you ate identified you as a follower of God?

Chapter 3

The Broken Plate
(How Man's Appetite Has Disconnected Him From God)

"Am I tough? Am I strong? Am I hard-core? Absolutely.

Did I whimper with pathetic delight when I sank my teeth into my hot fried-chicken sandwich? You betcha."

— James Patterson

From the beginning, our plate was a blessing. It was a plate of wonderful, natural delicacies with an endless supply of variety and sensation for our pallet. It was a plate of dependency that allowed us to experience the daily faithfulness of our Creator and Provider. It was a plate of distinction that set us apart as the masterpiece of God's creation. The plate of blessing, however, became a plate of brokenness.

The very first sin was food related. Imagine that. Adam and Eve didn't kill anyone. They didn't abuse one another or any animal. They didn't lie to one another or commit grand larceny. They simply went against God's one command of not eating one specific food. The sin was much deeper than the food, mind you. Certainly, the temptation was based on the serpent's appeal to "be like God", playing upon the lust of the flesh and the pride of life. He cunningly tied that to the one command that they were given and an appetite for both power and food, that seemed unquenchable. Eve took of the fruit and gave to her husband to eat. We see in this one act of disobedience several prevailing failures: the failure to trust God's word, the failure to deny temptation, the failure of a husband to not lead his wife, the failure to be honest with each other and God. And, all of this failure led to the plate of blessing becoming a plate of brokenness. All because they could not satiate their appetite with all that God had given them, but by giving in to the one thing, a piece of fruit, that God had kept from them. That one act of giving in to the human appetite is responsible for the entire curse upon all of creation as we know it. When you think about death, disease, heartache, despair, depression, thorns, thistles, child labor pains, and working by the sweat of your brow, you can thank one man and one piece of food. Everything that we know as painful and less than pleasant all started right here. The fall happens in Genesis 3:6. Notice the effects found in verses 17-19.

"And He said to Adam, 'Because you listened to your wife's voice and ate from the tree about which I commanded you, 'Do not eat from it': The ground is cursed because of you. You will eat from it by means of painful labor all the days of your life. It will produce thorns and thistles for you, and you will eat the plants of the field.'"

By the way I would like to interject the discovery that up until this point, all food was lush garden food. Now man is commanded to eat field food. What's the difference? "Garden food" is fresh fruits and vegetables full of antioxidants, vitamins, and minerals. "Field food" is wheat, barley, and grains, (bread) which we know still have vitamins and minerals, but has an entirely different make up that we have come to know as responsible for chronic levels of elevated insulin causing diabetes, cellular and arterial oxidation, and obesity. Could it be that this change in diet inadvertently led to the degradation of the human body that carried out the other curse, i.e. DEATH?

"You will eat bread by the sweat of your brow until you return to the ground, since you were taken from it. For you are dust, and you will return to dust." Genesis 3:19

Perhaps, among other lifestyle and planetary changes, God used an inferior diet as part of His curse of mortality.

Still don't think food is important to our connection to our Creator?

The curse of death brought about on mankind was tied to a change in diet. Consider 1 Corinthians 15:21-22a,

"For since death came through a man, the resurrection of the dead also comes through a man. For as in Adam all die..."

The curse that caused an eventual physical death on Adam was passed to all mankind, but even worse, a spiritual death, a disconnection from our Creator! The curse of sin through the eating of the fruit passed upon all people a nature of sin. Meaning, even when we are born without sin as innocent little babies, we are born in sin, having a natural affection to appease the human appetite of all things pleasurable even when not in God's will. This curse places us in direct opposition to a holy God who is just and righteous. We have lost our connectedness with the very One who created us and gave us life.

It didn't stop there, however. Food has played a huge role in our history of brokenness ever since. Not long after Noah, a man called righteous and upright, and his family came off the ark, he gives in to heavy drink, becomes intoxicated and caused a curse upon his son, Canaan. Food related sin. (Genesis 9)

Later we read (Genesis 25) of Esau who sold out his blessing and birthright to his brother Jacob for food, causing a major rift in the family and for generations to come. Essentially creating a biblical 'Hatfields and McCoys' situation. Food related sin.

When God steps in to free the Hebrew slaves from 400 years of slavery at the hands of Egypt, it doesn't take them long while enjoying their freedom to long for food of Egypt rather than God. (Exodus 16:3, Numbers 11:4, 5 & 21:5) Food related sin.

Lust of food brings a curse to the priest Eli's house.

"A man of God came to Eli and said to him, 'This is what the Lord says: 'Didn't I reveal Myself to your ancestral house when it was in Egypt and belonged to Pharaoh's palace? Out of all the tribes of Israel, I selected your house to be priests, to offer sacrifices on My altar, to burn incense, and to wear an ephod in My presence. I also gave your house all the Israelite fire offerings. Why, then, do all of you despise My sacrifices and offerings that I require at the place of worship? You have honored your sons more than Me, by making yourselves fat with the best part of all of the offerings of My people Israel.' Therefore, this is the declaration of the Lord, the God of Israel: 'Although I said your family and your ancestral house would walk before Me forever, the Lord now says, 'No longer! I will honor those who honor Me, but those who despise Me will be disgraced. Look, the days are coming when I will cut off your strength and the strength of your ancestral family, so that none in your family will reach old age. You will see distress in the place of worship, in spite of all that is good in Israel, and no one in your family will ever again reach old age. Any man from your family I do not cut off from My altar will bring grief and sadness to you. All your descendants will die violently. This will be the sign that will come to you concerning your two sons Hophni and Phinehas: both of them will die on the same day.'" 1 Sam 2:27-34

Whoa! God is no respecter of men, not even preachers! Could you imagine being the cause of such ancestral judgement because of your sacrilegious gluttonous ways? Food related sin.

And speaking of gluttony. That's a word that many preachers won't use. Drunken yes. Gluttony, well that's a word many shy away from. But why? What is it? Gluttony is simply overeating. But the Bible calls it a sin. As a matter of fact, the Bible puts gluttony on the same shelf as being drunk. You see, the sin of gluttony (and drunkenness) is like that of Adam's sin, it's self-control! The Bible calls gluttony a sin of the flesh and spirit; it's called the "god of the stomach." I believe we fall into hypocrisy by damning the drunkard for his overextension with alcohol while we stuff our faces with extra helping of mash potatoes. Yes, we have a problem. Let's not neglect to look at the beam in our own eye before acknowledging the speck in our brother's eye. We may be falling head long into a damning lifestyle of gluttony, and then making jokes and bragging about our church potluck dinners and how many plates we can put away. This must stop. This is food related sin at its best and it is destroying the testimony and image of the bride of Christ. Not only has food caused a disconnection between man and God, but now we see it causing a disconnect between the church and the world that He longs to save.

Chapter 4

The Blessed Plate
(How Food Connects to God)

"There is no love sincerer than the love of food."

— George Bernard Shaw, *Man and Superman*

Food should never be looked down upon. Like anything else, it is in how you approach it and how you use it. We have seen how damaging a bad approach can be. It has resulted in the downfall of the human race. It has been the subject of many curses and judgements throughout Bible and history. Even unto this day, it is a constant personal struggle of my own.

I was always a sickly child. I was skinny and full of ill health and allergies. I was also a very picky eater. You couldn't bribe me with a gold brick to eat vegetables. I didn't eat much, but what I did eat was processed and unhealthy. I don't blame my parents. They did the best they could, short of forcing good food down my throat. And, of course, they were not educated dietitians. They fed me the best food they knew how. We raised a garden, ate farm raised animals, and preserved as much as we could to keep us through the winter. By the time I was nine years old, I had my tonsils and adenoids removed. It was as if I could truly taste food for the first time in my life. I was finally able to taste! I mean really taste. And with this new ability, I did not let it go to waste. I indulged. Ok, I overindulged. I went from a skinny little runt to shopping in the "husky" section of the department store. I was an overweight kid with a complex. I hated my body and how I felt. I hated the husky section. Soon I hit high school and a growth spurt, and the weight came off. Then came college. During my sophomore year I ballooned back up. I had a horrible time with weight that lasted for another 10 years. Years of marriage, kids, and ministry kept me busy and I neglected my diet. That is, until I nearly died. By my late 20's I had exhausted by already unhealthy body and by burning the candle at both ends, I wrecked myself. I was sixty pounds overweight, tired, and in physical pain. My life quickly became depressed – I was empty.

My salvation didn't come from a fitness magazine, or health guru. By the time I had reached my end, a light had shown that offered a better way. It was this realization that God loves me regardless of how I feel about me. I did not need to perform for His love. I simply only needed to receive it. I needed to reconnect with my Savior through a relationship of grace and love. And so, I set forth on a journey of cleaning up my spiritual life, and THAT led to me cleaning up my plate, for which I found after all the brokenness I had endured because of how I approached food, was actually a plate of blessing.

I was given a renewed spirit. I felt free. But I was still fat. However, I began to see my body differently. I started seeing it as the temple of the Holy Spirit. "How could I put so much effort into my spiritual life, when it is so poorly reflected in my physical life?" I thought. And so, from my love for the Lord, I found a new love for my body in which I begin to learn and pay attention to. I began to clean up my plate and started exercising. I lost 60 pounds of fat that year (which I've kept off for eight years now!). I had a six- pack for the first time in my life! Most importantly, though, I discovered the beauty in food. I learned to treat food as it was intended, as a way to connect with my Creator, to enjoy fellowship with Him and others, and to fuel my body so that I am physically able to carry out His will for my life in this world. I found a love more sincere than a love for food.

Jesus the Foodie

Jesus Christ is known for many things: a carpenter, a rabbi, a healer, a prophet, and God incarnate.

But a foodie? What does a man who came to save the world have anything to do with food? Everything! Jesus, knowing quite well man's appetite for food and the history of Adam, used food as a bridge to reconnect man's understanding of his relationship with the Father. Consider how Jesus used the idea of food.

"'My food is to do the will of Him who sent Me and to finish His work,' Jesus told them." John 4:34

"Don't work for the food that perishes but for the food that lasts for eternal life, which the Son of Man will give you, because God the Father has set His seal of approval on Him." John 6:27

"'I am the bread of life,' Jesus told them. 'No one who comes to Me will ever be hungry, and no one who believes in Me will ever be thirsty again.'"
John 6:35

"But He answered, 'It is written: Man must not live on bread alone but on every word that comes from the mouth of God.'" Matthew 4:4

Jesus consistently connected our understanding of food and appetite for it to reveal His deeper truths and His true nature. As a matter of fact, other than language that was consistent with agricultural illustrations, food seems to be his greatest illustrator.

Jesus knew something else about food. More than being an easy way to connect people's understanding to His truth, it was a great way to connect people to him personally. It seems we almost constantly find Jesus attending dinner parties and eating with people in casual settings. We find him early on at the wedding in Cana in John chapter 2. Later he enjoys a very controversial dinner with sinners and a tax collector named Matthew, who became a disciple and the author of this narrative account in Matthew 9. In Luke 14 He uses a meal at a Pharisee's house as an opportunity to connect with the super religious and later in Luke 19, to connect with the least religious, a man named Zacchaeus. Often, He is found enjoying a meal with His own disciples, even broiling fish over a fire for them as an invitation to eat breakfast.

Jesus even used food to showcase His power and love for people; that His love and mercy is not only for their hearts, but their whole person. Hunger is a very real threat to the love that Jesus has for people. We see Him on two separate occasions performing a massive miracle in order to feed a massive crowd of hungry people, in Matthew 14 and Mark 8.

He takes hunger so seriously that He uses it as sort of a litmus test to validate those who are truly his followers and those who are not. In Matthew 25 we read of a time that will come when Jesus will separate out the believers from the non-believers by the way they treated "the least of these."

"For I was hungry and you gave Me something to eat; I was thirsty and you gave Me something to drink..." (verse 35a)

"Then the righteous will answer Him, 'Lord, when did we see You hungry and feed You, or thirsty and give You something to drink?'..." (verse 37a)

"And the King will answer them, 'I assure you: Whatever you did for one of the least of these brothers of Mine, you did for Me.'" (verse 40)

Yes, we are saved by grace through faith, but it is lived out through the way we love God and our neighbor! Food and drink are necessities of life. What a blessed way to live out our salvation from a God who has given us daily food, to give food to those who are without?

Jesus used food as the backdrop for, probably, the most controversial moments in His ministry. He didn't use it to garner more followers, but to test His real followers, resulting in thousands turning and walking away. Let me set up the scene. John chapter 6 starting in verse 25. Jesus and His disciples are enjoying a full day of teaching out in the open air. Thousands of men, women and children have heard of His healings and have ventured out to hear his words. The sermon goes long. There is concern. The disciples worry how they will feed these people. Jesus performs one of His greatest miracles by taking a small, donated lunch from a child, blesses it, and multiplies five loaves of bread and two fish. The abundance was so great that it feeds the whole crowd with an extra twelve baskets worth of leftovers to be collected! But, that's not controversial, that's just downright amazing. Wait for it...

Immediately He sends the disciples out in a boat into the Sea of Galilee. That night He walks to them on the water. But, while these amazing events are taking place, these people are in search. That was a tasty meal! Where can they find Him and get fed again? Finally, the next day, after traversing around the sea, they meet up with Him. But His reaction is less than appreciated.

"When they found Him on the other side of the sea, they said to Him, 'Rabbi, when did You get here?' Jesus answered, 'I assure you: You are looking for Me, not because you saw the signs, but because you ate the loaves and were filled. Don't work for the food that perishes but for the food that lasts for eternal life, which the Son of Man will give you, because God the Father has set His seal of approval on Him.'

'What can we do to perform the works of God?' they asked.

Jesus replied, 'This is the work of God — that you believe in the One He has sent.'

'What sign then are You going to do so we may see and believe You?" they asked. "What are You going to perform? Our fathers ate the manna in the wilderness, just as it is written: He gave them bread from heaven to eat'

Jesus said to them, 'I assure you: Moses didn't give you the bread from heaven, but My Father gives you the real bread from heaven. For the bread of God is the One who comes down from heaven and gives life to the world.'

Then they said, 'Sir, give us this bread always!'

'I am the bread of life,' Jesus told them. 'No one who comes to Me will ever be hungry, and no one who believes in Me will ever be thirsty again. But as I told you, you've seen Me, and yet you do not believe. Everyone the Father gives Me will come to Me, and the one who comes to Me I will never cast out. For I have come down from heaven, not to do My will, but the will of Him who sent Me. This is the will of Him who sent Me: that I should lose none of those He has given Me but should raise them up on the last day. For this is the will of My Father: that everyone who sees the Son and believes in Him may have eternal life, and I will raise him up on the last day.'

Therefore, the Jews started complaining about Him because He said, 'I am the bread that came down from heaven.' They were saying, 'Isn't this Jesus the son of Joseph, whose father and mother we know? How can He now say, 'I have come down from heaven?'

Jesus answered them, 'Stop complaining among yourselves. No one can come to Me unless the Father who sent Me draws him, and I will raise him up on the last day. It is written in the Prophets: And they will all be taught by God. Everyone who has listened to and learned from the Father comes to Me — not that anyone has seen the Father except the One who is from God. He has seen the Father. I assure you: Anyone who believes has eternal life. I am the bread of life. Your fathers ate the manna in the wilderness, and they died. This is the bread that comes down from heaven so that anyone may eat of it and not die. I am the living bread that came down from heaven. If anyone eats of this bread he will live forever. The bread that I will give for the life of the world is My flesh.'

At that, the Jews argued among themselves, 'How can this man give us His flesh to eat?'

So, Jesus said to them, 'I assure you: Unless you eat the flesh of the Son of Man and drink His blood, you do not have life in yourselves. Anyone who eats My flesh and drinks My blood has eternal life, and I will raise him up on the last day, because My flesh is real food and My blood is real drink. The one who eats My flesh and drinks My blood lives in Me, and I in him. Just as the living Father sent Me and I live because of the Father, so the one who feeds on Me will live because of Me. This is the bread that came down from heaven; it is not like the manna your fathers ate — and they died. The one who eats this bread will live forever'... From that moment many of His disciples turned back and no longer accompanied Him." (verses 25-58, 66)

What a turn of events! You would think, "Jesus, you have such an opportunity to create a huge group of followers! Chill out on the 'eat my flesh, drink my blood' stuff!" This, however unpopular, becomes a massively important moment in Jesus' ministry. Many have looked at this as mysterious and gross. Others dismissed it entirely. We can do neither. Was Jesus being literal about eating His flesh and drinking his blood? Yes. Sort of. See, there is a difference between "factually literal" and "metaphorically literal." I could say, "I am very hungry." That is factually literal. Or, I could say, "I could eat a horse!" That is metaphorically literal. Both carry the same idea. Jesus isn't expressing the need for cannibalism. He knew and understood that these people were more interested in the "thing" that they could get from Him, more than HIM. They wanted their bellies filled with more food. Food that would not last. Jesus is offering them a food that is eternal-Himself- that, in Him they would find a greater fulfillment and satiation, spiritually speaking. That His broken body and spilled blood would atone and suffice the wrath of God, bringing eternal salvation. That they would have to ingest and digest this sacrifice, accepting it as their payment for sins and salvation. "This bread" is a spiritual bread. "This bread" is Jesus who was born in Bethlehem, whose name translates to "house of bread."

It is interesting to see how the Lord used food, namely bread, to point to Himself. As pointed out before, bread, or grains, was a result of the curse upon creation through the fall of man into sin. I would point out a few more facts concerning this inferior food source.

First, grains when over consumed have the potential to lead to chronic health problems and diseases such as diabetes and heart disease. Christ, however, is the bread that heals.

Grains were a food that required man to work by the sweat of his brow in order to harvest and process it into food. Jesus is our bread of Sabbath rest, to give us rest for our souls as well as eternal rest in Him.

Grains and bread seem to never satiate. No matter how much you eat, it is hard to ever feel full, which leads to overeating. Jesus is the bread that satisfies completely.

Lastly, there is no such thing as an essential carbohydrate. Your body has the ability to produce its own glucose. Jesus is the essential Bread of Life that satisfies sin's curse and death's payment completely and fully.

I am not saying that bread or grains is bad. When consumed as a whole food in the proper amounts, it can be a part of a healthy balanced diet. I do believe that they are an inferior food when compared to fresh fruits and vegetables, and grass-fed or wild-caught meat. The inferiority of grains should be seen as an arrow that points us to our superior Bread of Jesus Christ. In doing so, we can appreciate a different, often overlooked asset that bread holds. Much like how the first Adam, who sinned, is able to point us to the last "Adam" who saved us from sin. Or, how that the Law, though good, was insufficient and unable to save us. But it possesses the ability and purpose of pointing to the New Covenant of grace. Bread is a perfect food source to point to Jesus!

The Communion: Food as a Way to Remember Christ's Death and Return

Imagine the evening before Jesus' arrest and crucifixion. This is a sacred, holy night. It is Passover.

Every Jew and their family are gathered around a sacred table of food that commemorates the Jew's exodus from their time as slaves in Egypt. Every morsel, every bite is a reminder of the bitterness of slavery and the sweetness of salvation. The paschal lamb is prepared. Jesus, with His disciples join in this sacred time of eating together but the atmosphere is tense. Jesus has washed their feet as a show of humility. He has reclined at the table. Everyone is dining. Jesus, knowing His time on earth is nearing its end chooses the most sacred thing in front of Him to encourage their hearts. The flickering flame of the oil lamps dance across their faces. Jesus reaches for the broken, pierced pieces of unleavened bread. Holding it up, He declares, "This is my body, broken for you. Take and eat it." Then, picking up the cup, "Drink from it, all of you. This is my blood of the covenant, which is poured out for many for the forgiveness of sins. I tell you, I will not drink from this fruit of the vine from now on until that day when I drink it new with you in my Father's kingdom."

The bread, being one of three pieces broken, that earlier in the meal, had been laid aside and wrapped in a white linen napkin. Three pieces signifying the trinity, the one broken and given to each. Jesus chose to use this as the deepest of illustrations to signify his death, burial and resurrection.

The wine. The blood of the new covenant of grace, poured out for the remission of sins on the world. The hope to come. A return of the blessed Redeemer, to redeem the fallen world through which one meal cursed...a new meal to save.

The Fast: Food as a Way to Hear From God

Fasting from food is as old as mankind itself. And, even though it has been around for centuries, it is still cloaked in mystery and misunderstanding. Many people see fasting as a way to express penance before the Lord for some sin or failure. I do not find this as any Biblical expectation. That would contradict God's grace extended through repentance, the turning away of sin. The need to punish our self is unnecessary. Christ took our punishment upon Himself while on the cross. God is not impressed by an act of short-term starvation in order to show your remorse.

Is fasting spiritual? Absolutely. Fasting, no matter for how long, gives the believer the ability to set aside time for prayer, meditation, and study. The act of devotion draws the heart of the believer to a more consecrated season, a season of focus and tenacity. Since, more often than not, a person who is fasting seems to pray more fervently than usual. And, as James reminds us in his 5th chapter, "The urgent request of a righteous person is very powerful in its effect" (verse 16b)

Fasting is often commanded in Scripture, especially during times when God's people need to see Him move or to have a great break though.

"Even now —this is the Lord's declaration —turn to Me with all your heart, with fasting ..." Joel 2:12a

"Isn't the fast I choose: To break the chains of wickedness, to untie the ropes of the yoke, to set the oppressed free, and to tear off every yoke?" Isaiah 58:6

"So we fasted and pleaded with our God about this, and He granted our request." Ezra 8:23

We see fasting carried out by men such as Moses, Elijah, Nehemiah, Daniel, and Jesus. The Pharisees even fasted twice a week!

I had never heard much preached on fasting growing up. Honestly, I didn't know anything about it. It wasn't until I was in college that I began to read what the Bible had to say about fasting. I was uneducated but eager. There was so much said about it in Scripture, it must be important. No one told me how to fast or how long to fast. So, I embarked upon my first fast with seven days in mind. For years afterwards, seven days seemed to be a staple timeline. Sometimes I would go shorter, maybe three or four days. There were times I would extend it by a week or two. But mostly I kept it at seven. I remember having some real breakthroughs. I grew closer to the Lord and more earnest in my spiritual disciplines. I'll tell you the truth though, I didn't always enjoy it. It was hard! I love food! To go seven days without eating was quite an ordeal. Usually by day three and four I would feel horrible! I suffered exhaustion, brain fog, aches, bad breath, and nausea. Often times, I would reach this point and tap out. "I've had enough. Surely the Lord didn't want me to go longer," I thought.

It was later, after I had reached good health in my early 30's that I finally realized what fasting was all about. I had researched a diet known as "keto" or "ketosis." During this time, I was researching and experimenting with different ways of eating in order to best optimize my health. I was dealing with a terrible auto-immune disorder that was very painful to live with and had no medical treatments.

Ketosis is the body's natural ability to switch from using glucose (the form of sugar in the blood stream) to using fat as a primary fuel source. When insulin lowers due to a lack of sugar in the blood, the body begins to break down body fat for fuel. The byproduct are molecules created in the liver called "ketones." Ketones are a wonderful fuel source for the body, especially the brain. What does all of this mean? Ketosis is the biological auxiliary fuel source during times of fasting! God did not want His followers suffering and dropping over dead because they stopped eating for a short period of time!

But even better, it's the benefits of being in ketosis that makes fasting easy, and beneficial!

When you are a carb burner--and most of you are--and you stop eating, your body has to make the metabolic shift to ketones. This takes a little bit of time and effort. During this time, your body dumps loads of electrolytes such as potassium, magnesium, sodium, chloride and calcium. And so, around day three or four you have depleted these electrolytes and are experiencing the "keto flu" – these feelings of brain fog and exhaustion. The following days as your body ramps up ketone production, you begin to feel great. Your hunger goes down, your energy goes up, your brain is operating clearer, and you feel like you can go weeks without eating. Which is exactly what I did. Now that I had become ketogenic by eating a diet that was very low in carbohydrates, moderate in protein, and high in fat, I decided to do a 30 day fast. My body was already in a simulated fasted state, being in ketosis. And, so I was able to start fasting without the hunger and keto flu. I fasted for 30 days, continuing my daily routines, uninterrupted, and even ran a 5k (3.2 miles) on day 30!

Now, I don't tell you this to brag, but simply to show you that God has given us the biological tools to use fasting as a way to draw closer to him, without hurting ourselves. And, if we learn how to use them, we can become more successful in fasting and praying.

Fasting is like the antenna on our old televisions. When the signal is coming in a bit fuzzy, we would adjust them until the signal came in clear. Often times, my prayer life seems a bit fuzzy and static. When your body goes into a fasted state and the brain begins to use ketones as fuel instead of glucose, the signal comes in clear. You can focus, recall, and retain information and thoughts like never before. Imagine your prayer life like that! It's the difference between using gasoline and rocket fuel.

We needn't decrease the spiritual side of fasting to understand the biological tools we are given that fasting is built for.

Aside from the biological purpose of fasting for spiritual reasons, we need to remember the health benefits. Fasting is the oldest medicine known to man. It has been used for centuries to treat sickness and disease of many types. When you fast, your body goes through a process known as "autophagy." Autophagy is a natural occurrence in the body wherein the body disassembles cells unnecessary or malfunctioning components. The body literally eats and disposes of unhealthy cells. This is a wonderful, natural detoxing process. The body will attack tumors, cancers, and diseased cells, leaving healthy cells to grow and multiply. When a cell is damaged, it creates free radicals in the body. These free radicals cause inflammation, oxidation, and disease. Some inflammation is good. When you cut your finger or bump your knee, your body signals white blood cells to the area and begins protecting and rebuilding the damage. You will notice swelling and redness. However, too much or prolonged inflammation will cause further breakdown of cells and tissues. This is very bad. When you fast, you send signals to your body that douses the fire of inflammation and takes out the trash of damaged cells. Thus, you will notice that after a few days of fasting, your hair, skin, and nails look and feel healthier. Your brain is shaper and clearer than before. Your aches and pains have diminished. I've seen skin tags on my clients fall off!

Our ancestors understood the benefits of feasting and fasting, and we should too. Food's role in our life is vital. It sustains us physically. We use its abundance to celebrate. We also use its absence to draw near to God and to grow in spirit and overall health.

The Fellowship: Food as a Way to Draw Closer as a Community of Faith

(Acts 2)

As I have pointed out, Jesus spent a great deal of time dining with people. Food has a way to nurture community. Perhaps it's a part of our nature to eat our meals with other people. We enjoy the relaxed atmosphere and conversation, and the joy of sharing tastes and foods. It has always been a part of the family to sit down together for a meal. There was a time when the Sunday meal was a big event and the extended family would gather together. For all major holidays and special occasions, we make it a point to surround it by a meal.

It should be no surprise then, that, as God created the local church and structured it according to spiritual growth and community building, He made eating together a part of it. Imagine the disciples and new believers after Jesus' resurrection. They were a tight knit community of religious outcasts who believed theirs was the mission of God. Remember, church is not a building. It is a community of believers, united in Christ to fulfill the great commission of making disciples of all nations. It is not a place to go, but a body to belong to. The word for "church" in the Greek is ecclesia, which means "called out ones." These who had been called out felt very different from the rest of the community. They were followers of Jesus. Often times ridiculed and persecuted for their faith, they had only one another to depend on. Their support came only from one another. They would bring in money at the beginning of each week that would help support one another and the poor.

Recently, I spent some time in China among the persecuted church. I believe they are living more closely to a first century model of church than anything I've ever seen before. With an atheist Communist government looming over them, constantly watching their every move and listening to their every word, even on their electronic devises, it has inadvertently created an "Acts" church. The believers speak in code. God is referred to as "Pops." Churches are referred to as "clubs." Pastors are simply "leaders." Cameras are everywhere. No, I mean it. Everywhere. The church's movements are decisive and intentional. More so, their relationships with one another are resolute. There is a sincere care for everyone. In America, many churches see those they attend with once or twice a week. We may have a monthly potluck meal for the sake of fellowship. In China, the dinner table is church. Without the ability to have their own church building where they can toll the bell and put out signs, they are finding that time together around mealtime is precious and unique. Meals become a place of sharing. Whether it be sharing of testimony or what Pops has been saying to them lately, or a time to express struggles and prayer needs, this time is holy and sanctified. It's also a time of celebration. The conversation is praiseworthy, while the atmosphere is jovial. They will order food that seems to never stop. In the center of the table, the food is placed on a wheel. The eldest of the table gets the honor of spinning the wheel throughout the night, as everyone reaches in with their chop sticks to sample each dish. This goes on for hours. Once they are finished, then begins the games. Eating games! The loser of each round has to take another bite. Which by this time seems a little gluttonous! And if they aren't foundering themselves on dumplings and fish, they are surely getting their fill of each other. The night wanes on and the mood changes. As things begin to settle down you can see in their eyes a fond realization of what they have really gathered for. This time is sacred. It 'could' be the last time they see each other. The leaders have already had conversations with their families with instructions of what to do if they are imprisoned. They know their small gathering could be broken up and dispersed at any moment. Time around the dinner table is holy.

Jesus believed this time was important as well. His first miracle was performed while attending a marriage ceremony in the small town of Cana. There he turned water into wine. Throughout His ministry He is accused of gluttony and drunkenness, not because He was guilty, but because He spent so much time in the context of eating and drinking. He would spot Zacchaeus in a tree and invite Himself to Zacchaeus' house for dinner. He would raise Lazarus from the dead and go to his house for food and celebration. He would meet and greet with sinners and tax collectors, only to find his way to their homes where they could lounge and eat together. After his resurrection He would join Himself with two depressed men walking home from Jerusalem to Emmaus. On the road he would explain the events they just witnessed by taking them through the teachings of the prophets, yet it was at the dinner table and the breaking of bread that they realized who He was. Also, after the resurrection, we can find Jesus appearing to His disciples while they bring in the evening catch from the sea, Jesus, hanging out on the beach broiling fish for them to eat. His conversation with them goes like this:

"Peter", he says. "Do you love me?"

"Yes, Lord, I love you," he says.

"Then feed my sheep."

Eating together as a church or community of faith should be an essential aspect of its function. Acts 2:42 tells us that the early church "broke bread from house to house." It doesn't mean that it is a special function, but that the function is special. Meaning, it doesn't have to be a separate or "special" event that is scheduled out and planned for on the church calendar. It is special enough that it should be enjoyed together as life...IN life. Church can happen around the dinner table on a regular basis. It can happen at your house or at your favorite restaurant. It can happen around a campfire or your local coffee shop. Jesus' incarnation dictated that, as a human, he would have to eat. That one thing that you do multiple times every day may be your greatest opportunity to connect to others and build communities of faith.

Chapter 5

The Believer's Plate
(How Christians Should Approach Food)

"If more of us valued food and cheer and song above hoarded gold, it would be a merrier world."
-- J.R.R. Tolkien

With Thanksgiving

I was raised in a southern fried, down home hospitable family that oozed values that may have seemed straight out of Mayberry. My mother would be in the kitchen preparing a meal large enough to feed an NFL football team. My dad would be catching up on the newest article from his hunting and fishing magazine, while my brother and I gathered dirt and all sorts of microbes underneath our fingernails outside playing. When everything was ready, that bugle call of "Boys!" would ring out from mom, alerting us that dinner was ready. We knew the routine. First stop, the bathroom to wash up. Next, we would grab our seats around the table, everyone in their places, as if we were actors taking our spots on stage, dad at the head of the table with mom to his right. My brother and I would square up, adjacent and ready to dive into mom's savory dishes. Hats off. Ready? Not quite. We knew better than to reach in before there was a blessing over the food. It was often a draw. Who offered thanks for our meal usually fell to me, probably because I was just ready to eat. And if submitting to be the demand of tradition got me closer to eating, then that was all right by me.

It seems as though you don't see many bowed heads around the dinner table these days. Is it simply a tradition of the past? Has it gone the way of Mayberry? Still living in the South, I can occasionally spot a couple or a family take a moment to pray over their meal. It stands out. It's definitely not the norm. We live in a fast-paced culture in which we scarf down our food and give little to no thought about what we are eating, let alone where it came from. Even in my own time of thanksgiving, it has at times, become ritualistic at best. My prayer might sound something like, "Dear Lord, thank you for this food. I pray you bless it to the nourishment of my body. In Jesus' name. Amen" Commence chow down.

We need to take a fresh look at eating with thanksgiving. We need to see it more than a tradition or routine. As we approach food, if we do so with sincere thanksgiving, it will change our lives.

Perhaps the earliest recorded practice of giving thanks for your meal comes from the Old Testament command of Deuteronomy 8:10 that says,

"When you eat and are full, you will praise the Lord your God for the good land He has given you."

Continuing with this command, we see it exemplified by the Lord, Himself.

"'But we only have five loaves and two fish here,' they said to Him.

'Bring them here to Me,' He said. Then He commanded the crowds to sit down on the grass. He took the five loaves and the two fish, and looking up to heaven, He blessed them. He broke the loaves and gave them to the disciples, and the disciples gave them to the crowds. Everyone ate and was filled." Matthew 14:17-20

"He took the seven loaves and the fish, and He gave thanks, broke them, and kept on giving them to the disciples, and the disciples gave them to the crowds." Matthew 15:36

"As they were eating, Jesus took bread, blessed and broke it, gave it to the disciples, and said, 'Take and eat it; this is My body.'" Matthew 26:26

"Then He took the five loaves and the two fish, and looking up to heaven, He blessed and broke the loaves. He kept giving them to His disciples to set before the people." Mark 6:41

"It was as He reclined at the table with them that He took the bread, blessed and broke it, and gave it to them." Luke 24:30

Approaching your meal with reverence and blessing is further taught by the Apostle Paul.

"If I partake with thanks, why am I slandered because of something I give thanks for? Therefore, whether you eat or drink, or whatever you do, do everything for God's glory." 1 Corinthians 10:30, 31

"Whoever observes the day, observes it for the honor of the Lord. Whoever eats, eats for the Lord, since he gives thanks to God; and whoever does not eat, it is for the Lord that he does not eat it, yet he thanks God." Romans 14:6

"For everything created by God is good, and nothing should be rejected if it is received with thanksgiving." 1 Timothy 4:4

Perhaps food provides an honest and telling look at the gratitude of our heart. I live in a community that has a large amount of homeless men and women. Our community does well to look after and meet the needs of thee desperate people. One of the local ministries called "The Least of These" provides breakfast every Saturday morning from a downtown parking lot, along with handing out clothing and prayers said. The first time I joined in to help, I was immediately drawn to the attitude of gratitude these people had shown. As lines formed to make their way to enjoy scrambled eggs, bacon, and pancakes, individuals would bow their heads and give thanks. One gentleman took it upon himself to loudly declare his gratitude as a representative of the group. To whom many of them were praying, I don't know. Their prayers were silent and personal. Regardless, the overwhelming sense of thanksgiving and gratitude was immense. These people knew this meal was a blessing, a blessing for which they may not see again for a while. Their next meal could be days later, possibly from a dumpster or trash can. I have found that thanksgiving for food often follows times of want. The flip side of that, however, is that during times of abundance, our gratitude seems to wane. How soon we forget what a great blessing food is when our refrigerators and pantries are stuffed full. We know that if we run low on some groceries, we can simply run by a large box grocery store and choose from more food choices than most people will see in their lifetime in many places around the world. How many times have you given thanks for your local farmer? Have you ever stopped outside of your local grocery to give God glory for the abundance of ready to eat food? We don't have to wait for the harvest, we live in it daily!

Did you know that there is a physiological importance to approaching food with thanksgiving? There is an old saying which states "you are what you eat."

That's not necessarily true. In reality, you are what you absorb. Our health is reflected in the nutrients that our body breaks down and absorbs from the food we eat. Many of us are hurried as we grab our next bite, barely chewing sufficiently before we swallow, and moving about on to our next task before we have had time to digest. Here is where thanksgiving and gratitude become really cool. If we pause to reflect and offer thanksgiving before we eat, our body reacts accordingly. Simply consider, as you look upon the food that has been prepared, you take a moment to give thanks for the animal whose life was given in order to feed you. Consider and give thanks for the farmer who grew and harvested your vegetables. Stop and give thanks to the Lord for His great provision and abundance, asking him to bless this food before you. As all of that sounds spiritual, and it is, there is something biological taking place as well. During this moment of gratitude, signals are sent to the brain, which sends messages to the body. Levels of neurotransmitters such as serotonin, GABA, and dopamine rise, giving you the feeling and sensation of joy, peace, and pleasure. This avenue of messengers between the brain and the gut, called the gut brain axis, is vitally important for the break down and absorption of nutrients. It calms your nervous system and sets the body up for "rest and digest." Stomach acids are produced and smooth digestive muscles can relax allowing for peristalsis, the involuntary constriction and relaxation of the muscles of the intestines and intestinal canals, creating wave-like movements that pushes food through these canals. While you are exercising gratitude, your digestive system is reaping the benefits of being able to function in a safe and relaxed state. This is to your benefit! You get to enjoy your food, without the uncomfortable feelings of being bloated and the aggravation of acid reflux. Also, because you are able to more properly and slowly digest your food, you reap a greater yield of nutrients that will give you more energy, brain function and overall better health. And friend, that is something to be thankful for!

With Unbelievers and the Weak in Mind

Our relationship with food can actually affect our relationship with others in tremendous ways. When I say tremendous, I mean we can tremendously help or tremendously hurt their relationship with us, and even more so, their relationship with God. So little thought is ever given to this idea, yet the Bible is explicit here. Jesus was accosted by the religious for his casual dining with "sinners," and yet, by sinners, He was celebrated for this. He offended people when His disciples neglected to wash their hands before eating. He was accused of blasphemy by the Pharisees while doing a little grocery shopping during the Sabbath.

"On the Sabbath He was going through the grain fields, and His disciples began to make their way picking some heads of grain. The Pharisees said to Him, 'Look, why are they doing what is not lawful on the Sabbath?'

He said to them, 'Have you never read what David and those who were with him did when he was in need and hungry — how he entered the house of God in the time of Abiathar the high priest and ate the sacred bread — which is not lawful for anyone to eat except the priests — and also gave some to his companions?' Then He told them, 'The Sabbath was made for man and not man for the Sabbath. Therefore, the Son of Man is Lord even of the Sabbath.'" Mark 2:23-2b

Jesus used food as a teaching moment for the "religious elite" to show them the error of their theology. It certainly brought about quite an offense. Yet, we know Jesus came to "make straight the way" that the Pharisees had twisted. Often times, in our own religious circles we get ourselves hemmed up into debate over what is right and what is wrong when it comes to eating. The argument is always based in law and man's righteousness; his attempt to appease God through food and drink. I imagine there is occasion for the believer to enact some controversy in order to make a point that points to true theology of God's grace and freedom in Christ, though I would caution you to be prayerful, full of wisdom and discernment here. It is not our right to debate or wrangle about traditions and vain arguments that further lead to division and offense. I think it best that we point to Scripture and Christ when Christian legalists try to condemn you for what you eat and drink.

"Accept anyone who is weak in faith, but don't argue about doubtful issues. One person believes he may eat anything, but one who is weak eats only vegetables. One who eats must not look down on one who does not eat, and one who does not eat must not criticize one who does, because God has accepted him." Romans 14:1-3

"Therefore, don't let anyone judge you in regard to food and drink or in the matter of a festival or a new moon or a Sabbath day. These are a shadow of what was to come; the substance is the Messiah." Colossians 2:16-17

We should pay much attention to those who do not believe. Our greatest desire in life should be to see people come to know Jesus Christ as Lord and Savior of their life, to glorify the grace of God. With that in mind, everything that we say and do should be for that purpose, and not to damage it. So, let me build my case.

First, we have freedom in Christ. With that freedom comes the allowance of eating things that once was prohibited to His people, the Israelites. I can tell you I am thankful for Jesus every time I eat a plate of pulled pork BBQ! My righteousness is not found in what I eat or abstain from eating. My righteousness is only found in the blood and sacrifice of Jesus Christ.

Secondly, with that kind of freedom comes a great deal of responsibility. What I am free to do may not always be what is best to do. The Apostle makes this case in 1 Corinthians 6:12, 13:

"Everything is permissible for me, but not everything is helpful. Everything is permissible for me, but I will not be brought under the control of anything. Food for the stomach and the stomach for food, but God will do away with both of them."

And, also 1 Corinthians 10:23,24,

"Everything is permissible, but not everything is helpful. Everything is permissible, but not everything builds up. No one should seek his own good, but the good of the other person."

When we are eating in the company of an unbeliever, we should use this as a litmus test. Does what I am eating and drinking build up, or tear down? "I have freedom here, but do I have edification?"

You may be asking the question, "How does food have any effect on building up or tearing down a person's faith?" Perhaps it's not so much of their faith that is being affected as it is your testimony, which may be the cause or casualty of their faith. There are different reasons why. Let's consider just a few.

Cultural differences are tricky. You were raised to eat and drink certain things. Because of that, it is normal, and you give very little thought. To you, it is not weird or gross. If you are American, there is hardly anything more culturally traditional than a hotdog. You probably eat it with no thought whatsoever that that might be seen as strange, peculiar, or even gross to another culture. I mean, do you know what a hotdog is made out of? Yuk! Okay, but consider the fact that what another deems normal, you deem gross and off limits. When you are hosted by someone that is from another culture (or even just a bad cook), it is impolite and sometimes a great offense to reject what has been offered. When I went into ministry years ago, I prayed a prayer saying, "Lord, if you will keep it down, I will eat it." I have never wanted to offend my host. There have been some questionable moments and really awful food! I have remained faithful to my promise and the Lord has remained faithful on His end. On my recent trip to Beijing, this was put to this test. I had a feeling I would encounter some strange foods. I made it a point to not ask what I was eating until after I had successfully eaten it! I am honest when I say it was some of the best food I've ever eaten, and my Chinese hosts were most pleased by my appreciation of cow intestine, squid, and goat testicle. You may find yourself in a situation that what is sitting before you is "weird" and "gross." Remember, to your host, it is normal and delicious, and their aim is to please you. It is better to stomach it and save face and your witness.

Religious and moral issues are something that we need to be very sensitive about. As a believer, you do not want to practice something that goes against your convictions or the will of God. A food sacrificed to idols is obviously off limits. So, how do we navigate this issue?

"About eating food offered to idols, then, we know that an idol is nothing in the world, and that there is no God but one. For even if there are so-called gods, whether in heaven or on earth — as there are many "gods" and many "lords"—yet for us there is one God, the Father. All things are from Him, and we exist for Him. And there is one Lord, Jesus Christ. All things are through Him, and we exist through Him.

However, not everyone has this knowledge. In fact, some have been so used to idolatry up until now that when they eat food offered to an idol, their conscience, being weak, is defiled. Food will not make us acceptable to God. We are not inferior if we don't eat, and we are not better if we do eat. But be careful that this right of yours in no way becomes a stumbling block to the weak. For if someone sees you, the one who has this knowledge, dining in an idol's temple, won't his weak conscience be encouraged to eat food offered to idols? Then the weak person, the brother for whom Christ died, is ruined by your knowledge. Now when you sin like this against the brothers and wound their weak conscience, you are sinning against Christ. Therefore, if food causes my brother to fall, I will never again eat meat, so that I won't cause my brother to fall." 1 Corinthians 8:4-13

What is an idol to you? Nothing. You know there is no God but God. Yet, knowing that this food is offered, Paul warns us to be careful with this knowledge. Proceeding without taking into account one weak in the faith or an unbeliever may affect their faith negatively. Their assumption is that you are sanctioning food offered to idols. If your Buddhist host has offered his food to one of his gods, and you know about it, and he knows you know about it, and then you eat it, he perceives what he has done is good and acceptable. This is not good.

"Eat everything that is sold in the meat market, asking no questions for conscience' sake, for the earth is the Lord's, and all that is in it. If one of the unbelievers invites you over and you want to go, eat everything that is set before you, without raising questions of conscience. But if someone says to you, 'This is food offered to an idol,' do not eat it, out of consideration for the one who told you, and for conscience' sake. I do not mean your own conscience, but the other person's. For why is my freedom judged by another person's conscience? If I partake with thanks, why am I slandered because of something I give thanks for?

Therefore, whether you eat or drink, or whatever you do, do everything for God's glory. Give no offense to the Jews or the Greeks or the church of God, just as I also try to please all people in all things, not seeking my own profit, but the profit of many, so that they may be saved." 1 Corinthians 10:25-33

I remember a time that my Executive Pastor and I were building a relationship with a young Indian family who had moved into our community. They were very devout Hindu. We loved them with a great tenacity and did our best to serve them well. Our small town had limited food for people wanting to prepare Indian cuisine. One day, he and I were going into the city to shop at a large world grocery store and we thought of our Indian friends. I called to see if they would like us to pick up any food for them while we were out. "Two apricots," he said. Later that week when I saw him and asked how they had enjoyed their apricots, he said, "Oh no, they were not for eating. My wife used them for sacrifice." My ministry cohort and I had a good laugh, figuring we just unknowingly aided and abetted idol worship! Sometimes ignorance is bliss.

I've also dealt with situations that were moral issues, not religious. It seems diet has become as hot a subject as politics and religion. Everyone sees their diet as the "right diet." No more so, that I've found, as with the vegan community. Vegans, probably, more than anyone else, have tied morality into their diets, in which I applaud to an extent. I firmly agree that food should be ethically raised and harvested, but that goes for animals as well as vegetables. I believe we have allowance and examples throughout Scripture for eating flesh. I love meat. I eat it every day. My belief that I was created to have dominion over animals with the allowance and benefits of harvesting and eating makes me a happy omnivore. But my vegan friends disagree with me. I have two vegan friends that I love and adore. They do not know the Lord and their worldview is a secular, non-Christian worldview. They view the world and their diet through different lenses. I want them to know the love and freedom of Jesus and so it is important to me to spend time with them. They know that I love them. When they come to my house, they get to eat a very well prepared, delicious vegan meal. I am happy, for that moment, eating vegetables cooked in coconut oil, with seeds, nuts, and fruit. I want to be mindful and sensitive to what is important to them. Going to such an extent to show that has won me great trust and rapport with my friends.

With whom and where you eat may be just as important. It seems Jesus took great steps to eat in the right places with the right people. How often we would see Him eating and dining with the ill repute.

"Then Levi hosted a grand banquet for Him at his house. Now there was a large crowd of tax collectors and others who were guests with them. But the Pharisees and their scribes were complaining to His disciples, 'Why do you eat and drink with tax collectors and sinners?' Jesus replied to them, 'The healthy don't need a doctor, but the sick do. I have not come to call the righteous, but sinners to repentance.'" Luke 5:31, 32

"One Sabbath, when He went to eat at the house of one of the leading Pharisees, they were watching Him closely." Luke 14:1

"All the tax collectors and sinners were approaching to listen to Him. And the Pharisees and scribes were complaining, 'This man welcomes sinners and eats with them!'" Luke 15:1, 2

"The Son of Man has come eating and drinking, and you say, 'Look, a glutton and a drunkard, a friend of tax collectors and sinners!'" Luke 7:34

Jesus intentionally placed Himself in an atmosphere that He could associate with sinners and be seen doing so. Typically, we find Jesus in even the most intimate of settings, their homes! The Pharisees view of Jesus' actions was "guilty by association." "If He eats with them, He must be one of them." Granted, you and I know that we are ALL sinners, including the Pharisees, and that Jesus was completely innocent of any and all sins. This perception is, however, important. We need to let food and dining create an even playing field. It needs to knock down walls. Eating with people of differing socio-economic status, or race, or background…these present a witness to the world that we (and Jesus) are for all people.

He did not, however, put Himself into places that may have caused unnecessary controversy. I believe the home is the best place to entertain, whether yours or theirs. I believe next to that is the public square, a restaurant or some other dining venue. I do not believe it is ever necessary to venture into a place that could cause an occasion for stumbling. Though permissible, is it beneficial to go to the bar or club? Be cautious here. Use prayer and wisdom. You want to win strippers to the Lord? Great! Should you go to the strip club to do it? Probably not. Take Christ's example and follow it. They may have sought to accuse Him, but they could not convict Him. Be blameless.

With Self-Control

We should never approach anything that is sacred haphazardly. When I say that I immediately think of things like prayer, worship, baptism, communion, and other spiritual practices that have been sanctified or set apart by God. But, is food any different? You've already seen how important food has been in establishing dependency on God, an identity in God, and a renewed covenant with God. All of these factors alone should teach us that food and the act of eating is sacred. And if that's not enough, consider the life sustaining importance of this act; meaning, if you don't, you die! That, in and of itself makes eating sacred. But are we too cavalier? Are we too thoughtless and reckless when it comes to approaching food?

My how times have changed. My grandparents' wisdom sounded like a broken record. "Waste not, want not." For a generation who grew up through and survived the Great Depression of the 1930's, they learned how valuable every morsel of food was. That meal of cornbread and beans may not have been the most appetizing of meals, certainly when it was on its third or fourth go around as leftovers. But it was all they may have had, and the possibility was real, it may be the last they might have for a while. This scarcity made their food even more sacred. Wasting it was not an option. We live in such a time of abundance that I fear food has lost its sacredness. The amount of wasted food on a daily basis from the average household could feed a small country. I see children pushing their unwanted chicken tenders and fries away from them, snubbing their meal uninterested, but mesmerized by the small tiny cheap toy that accompanied it. The so called "value meal" then gets thrown in the trash where it will be discarded and considered unfit to eat.

On the flip side of that is a word that we tend to shy away from: gluttony. It's typically a word that doesn't even appear in our vernacular. We heard about it, perhaps, in World Civilization class in school. The Romans were known for their gluttony. If there was one thing the Romans prized more than the human body, it was the food that went into it. A Roman party or festival would not be complete without an abundance of food. These guys knew how to eat. Let me rephrase that. These guys knew how to gorge! They would eat and drink all day and all through the night. They weren't just good at eating, but they were good at purging as well. Could you imagine eating so much food that you had to vomit just so that you could continue eating? That is gluttony.

Gluttony is still a problem today. We may not practice it in the same ways as the Romans, but it is a problem nonetheless. Let me cast some light upon what it means to commit gluttony. Some would see it as simply overeating. It's a bit more complicated than that. At the heart of gluttony, or the act of overeating, is another issue. A greater issue. Self-control. For most, if not all people, gluttony is caused by a lack of self-control. I grew up mastering the technique of the loss of self-control and committing gluttony. I was taught to "clean my plate." Meaning, eat everything on my dinner plate, leaving no food to waste. "Waste not, want not," right? So, my brain would never shut off or send the signal to my gut to stop eating, not until all the food on my plate was gone. And have you ever noticed, though, that portion sizes have grown quite substantially? I've been cleaning my plate for years, and the plate has gotten larger!

Gluttony has definite consequences that the majority of Americans and many people around the world are reaping. The obvious is obesity. Our society, our generation is the fattest generation in all of American history. It has become so common now that the World Health Organization calls it an epidemic. That means it's large and spreading, just like our midsections. With the rising levels of obesity also comes the rising levels of heart disease and diabetes, which are currently listed in the top ten as causes for death in the World.

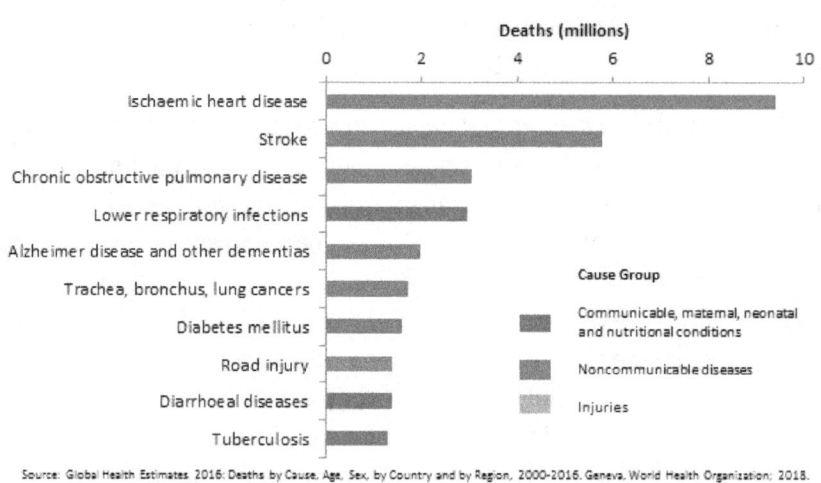

(1)

Other causalities stemming from gluttony would be childhood obesity, joint replacement, and a lack of overall quality of life. People are eating more, growing more, and moving less. Energy levels are dropping as the numbers on the scale go up.

But let me draw your attention to, what I believe, is a greater problem with gluttony. It is a sin. Simple as that. It is against the will of God! As seen in the very first sin, the rebellion of man against God, it was a matter of self-control to eat something that was not permitted. And yet, it is commonplace in our lives. At this point some of you are going to grow uncomfortable and perhaps label me a legalist. Well, I'm not going to sugar coat it...you may eat that too! Okay, that joke was harsh, but so is the reality of what we are doing. It is NOT okay to rebel against the will and authority of God, openly and knowingly, and disregard it as a joke. In my own denomination camp, we often joke about gluttony, bragging about our potluck dinners, where we have an entire table set aside for desserts. Where you're not done eating until you are carrying two, three, or even four empty paper plates to the trash can, smiling and joking about how good that was. Gluttony put Jesus on the cross and we joke about it. And worse, we prod and jab, and tempt others, "Oh, come on, eat up!" or "Come on, what's one more brownie?!" Once, after I had spent years overcoming food addiction and weight problems, a man at a church potluck came up behind me and shoved an entire plate of desserts under my nose and chided me to indulge, seeming almost offended if I didn't. Would we put a bottle of whiskey out and tempt a recovered or recovering alcoholic to drink? Of course not! The comparison is the same.

The Bible makes no distinction between gluttony and drunkenness.

"They will say to the elders of his city, 'This son of ours is stubborn and rebellious; he doesn't obey us. He's a glutton and a drunkard.'"
Deuteronomy 21:20

"For the drunkard and the glutton will become poor, and grogginess will clothe them in rags."
Proverbs 23:21

"Let us walk with decency, as in the daylight: not in carousing and drunkenness; not in sexual impurity and promiscuity; not in quarreling and jealousy. But put on the Lord Jesus Christ, and make no plans to satisfy the fleshly desires." Romans 13:13-14

Drunkenness and gluttony are essentially the same thing. The root, or the seed, is the same: self-control. When one lacks self-control with an alcoholic drink, their body reacts to the overabundance and we call it drunkenness. Similarly, when we lack the same self-control with food, our body reacts to the overabundance with negative effects. I've never been drunk on alcohol. That is true. I've been "food drunk" plenty. I've eaten myself into a sickly stupor. I've eaten so much in one sitting, I felt groggy and lethargic. I couldn't move! My body had to deal with the excess insulin and the massive work of digestion. When a person drinks too much alcohol, their liver is not capable of metabolizing it, causing the alcohol to run free in the blood stream, impairing their motor skills and health. When a person eats too much food, the pancreas and insulin response is not capable of keeping up with it, and thus high amounts of glucose are allowed to float freely in the blood, also, impairing motor skills and health. Think of gluttony as "foodalism." Before we judge an individual for being an alcoholic, we may need to deal with us being a foodaholic. A person can overcome this by producing the Spiritual fruit of self-control.

We must practice self-control when we approach food. We must be able to distinguish what is necessary and unnecessary portions. Every person has what's called a basal metabolic rate. The basal metabolic rate is the rate at which the body burns energy at rest that is required to live. We can increase our calorie consumption based on our activity level and need for more calories. Anything more than that is unnecessary and unhealthy. I'm not saying that everyone needs to start counting calories, but I want you to understand, your body needs a certain amount, and then that's it. Have the self-control that allows you to be able to eat what you need and be satisfied. Be prepared. That will probably not allow you to finish your plate. This will be like drug recovery for many people. They have wired their brains to eat so much extra food, and even the wrong types of food, that it has caused addiction and craving. Self-control is essential.

And then lastly, but certainly most importantly, we need to come to the realization that gluttony is a form of idolatry. You've probably never imagined that food could be considered an idol. Idolatry is the act of placing anything in place of the love, faith, and authority of God in our life. When Jesus was asked by His disciples to teach them to pray, He mentions food.

"Therefore, you should pray like this: Our Father in heaven, Your name be honored as holy. Your kingdom come. Your will be done on earth as it is in heaven. Give us today our daily bread." Matthew 6:9-11

This model prayer teaches us to establish a relationship with God (Our Father), to start with praise (Your name be honored as holy), and to express His will (Your kingdom come and will be done). The very first request given as a model for us to pray is a request of food. (Give us today our daily bread). This daily request of food takes us back to Eden, when man was solely dependent upon God to supply his every meal. This request is beckoning God to be our "Jehovah Jireh," or God provider. It establishes Him as the source and provider of our daily sustenance. When is the last time you prayed a daily prayer asking God to feed you? Or has your faith been placed in what is common, abundant, and readily available? Do we even need to trust in God's provision for food? Is our trust more in a full refrigerator and pantry? Or a regular paycheck to purchase food? This was a hard lesson learned by the children of Israel during a time that God wanted to teach them His everlasting faithfulness in earthly provision. When they complained about not having food, he sent food from Heaven. His instructions were clear in Exodus 16:16.

Every morning you will find manna. Only collect enough for the day. An omer. Fill it for you and your family.

For every family who tried to store away more, by the next morning, it had rotted and collected maggots. God is saying, "I am your God. I will provide what you need. You don't need to be a glutton!" We may have an abundance of food, but we should continually seek our Heavenly Father as our provider, recognizing that every morsel is given by His hand.

"Don't become idolaters as some of them were; as it is written, 'The people sat down to eat and drink, and got up to play.'" 1 Corinthians 10:7

This verse describes an attitude of mindless and inconsiderate disregard for the Provider. We are reminded of a people who are just there for the food. The act of eating and drinking became more important than the One providing it.

"Their end is destruction; their god is their stomach; their glory is in their shame." Philippians 3:19a

So many of us are led by our appetite for fleshly things. We are led by our stomachs. Our stomachs have become our gods. Our idols. From a spiritual perspective, to deal with the root sin, is no different than any other sin. Confession and repentance. We must cast down our idols. Perhaps the love of food is your idol. Confess it and cast it down. Gluttony is a heart issue, not a stomach issue. What is it that has your heart? Chocolate? Pizza? Sugar? Steak? Pray to God and ask forgiveness. Go on a fast of these foods to help detach the addiction. Reestablish an attitude of sacredness with food and the act of eating. Start to see it as an act of honor and worship to God. Eat only what you need without wasting.

"Therefore, brothers, by the mercies of God, I urge you to present your bodies as a living sacrifice, holy and pleasing to God; this is your spiritual worship. Do not be conformed to this age, but be transformed by the renewing of your mind, so that you may discern what is the good, pleasing, and perfect will of God." Romans 12:1, 2

With Quality Control

Have you ever heard of a health food store? Does that even make sense? What then does that make every other food store?

I admit, I was raised with certain advantages. I was a farm kid. Much of our food was raised or grown by our own hands. We had an intimate and special relationship with our food. I can remember the start of every spring as my dad would plow and till the garden. The ground cover that we sowed in the fall would be turned over by the plow where it would decompose and provide nutrients for the new seeds. I loved the final till of the ground. It made the dirt soft and powdery. My brother and I would run and jump in our bare feet leaving tracks as if it was a fresh coat of new snow. This was the time that the work began. We set out lines that would mark the rows. And row by row, section by section, we planted seeds that would provide beans, corn, broccoli, cauliflower, peppers, watermelon, cantaloupe, zucchini, cucumbers, carrots, and potatoes. As the tender young plants made their way out of the ground, it was my brother's and my job to weed the garden with a hoe. I hated that job. We composted our plants, put up deer fence to keep hungry, invasive wildlife out. We took great care to make sure our plants had all they needed in order to produce high quality food. Even though I despised the work as a kid, having to spend perfectly good summer days that I could've been playing ball with my friends, instead shucking truckloads of corn, picking and snapping beans, and digging up potatoes, I appreciate that we always had homegrown, nutrient dense food on our table.

I remember helping my parents slaughter hogs and package the hams that would hang in the barn for country ham, or curing out bacon and chitterlings, also known as chitlins. If you're not from the American South, you probably don't know what a chitlin is. It is similar to a pork rind, but with the skin, and deeeeelicious! I collected eggs from a hen house and watched my father scald and pluck chicken feathers. We had a yearly supply of venison and wild game such as deer, squirrel, rabbit, turtle, and freshwater fish. Our beef was grass-fed and pasture raised. The term "organic" was unheard of. All of our food was organic.

You probably grew up differently. By the turn of the 19th century, many Americans still had connection to agriculture. Small, sustainable farms were seen dotting the American landscape. Supermarket food was fresh. Local butchers still had business on Main Street, where you could go and order your fresh cut of meats. Those days are long gone. And with them, the quality of America's (and much of the world's) food supply. With people's livelihoods becoming ever more urban-centric, there is more demand on factory farmed and factory produced food. Food has become an industry. Industry is based on commerce, money. In a supply and demand relationship, we need food…and the companies (not farmers) have what we need.

As food has become industrialized and monetized, it has become a marketable product. Doesn't that sound strange? Food is marketed? Food is necessary, why does it need marketing? Because companies are competing for your money! Reread that statement. You are a consumer of their goods. In this dog-eat-dog world, it takes tactics of competition to win. You're probably thinking of packaging, right? Sure, food packaging is a huge part of marketing. Companies hire marketing consultants that base their advertising on proven science that uses color, images, lettering, and placement to attract and draw your attention to their product. Let's look at some of these.

Betty Crocker is the queen of easy, quick fix, desserts from a box. Once upon a time, you would buy eggs, flour, sugar, salt, baking soda, and a few other ingredients, spend precious time mixing, measuring, and baking to produce a cake, or cookies. By the 1950's, housewives were joining their husbands in the workforce, leaving very little time to prepare such desserts. In walks Betty Crocker (figuratively speaking), and a solution. Pick up your favorite cake mix and within minutes, your pre-mixed ingredients are turned into a beautiful "homemade" dessert. Hey, if it's good enough for Betty it's got to be good enough for us! Here's the problem. Betty Crocker is a fictional character created by a marketing team to purport an image geared toward enticing you, not to buy a cake, but to buy into an idea: packaged, ready or near ready-made food and no need to feel guilty about it.

Companies have created identities to represent their foods for decades. Some, like Aunt Jemima, have fictitiously been created to give us a personal or intimate relationship with the product. Others like Colonel Sanders, Sara Lee, and Chef Boyardee serve as inviting faces that validate the supposed goodness and "home cooked" feel of their product.

They worked even harder to entice children. Growing up as an 80's kid, I remember the public service announcements and campaigns run by First Lady Nancy Reagan, telling us kids to "Just Say No" to drugs. Everywhere were warnings of talking to strangers and steering clear of unsafe and suspicious places and people. The 80's really did set up the "overly protective" parents of the 90s! But they left out food advice. Adversely, we were the intentional targets, the bullseye, of food marketers. Our pancake syrup bottle, Mrs. Butterworth, assured us her sweet sugary syrup was delicious. I sure did love Mrs. Butterworth. Why would a sweet, sincere pancake syrup bottle like that lie to me, anyway? Fast food restaurants created boxed meals for kids, loaded with games, puzzles, and toys. As a matter of fact, and I will admit this now, I chose the cereal I wanted based on the cartoon character that represented it and the toy that they offered inside. One cereal in particular was a disgusting, dry, and tasteless mouthful of processed corn. I had to have it. Inside of that box was a custom license plate for my BMX bike that was sure to make me the coolest kid on my street. Who cares if what was I eating tasted like cardboard!

Why do companies feel so compelled to spend so much time, energy, and money to sell something that we already need? As mentioned before, there is the need to sell the 'idea' of eating food from a factory or processing plant. And that has been sold. The other cause is the need to sell garbage and label it as food.

Our food is no longer food. It's mostly processed junk, void of nutrients and anything natural. The cost to grow, package, ship, and sell fresh natural food to the billions of people who need it is seen as too costly and implausible. Now that they have accepted the idea of eating food that comes from a factory and in a box, we are now embracing that what we are eating is 'normal' and good. On the contrary. Today, food manufacturers are hard at work in their laboratories, creating additives, flavors, colors, and textures that will appeal to your senses and mask the desire for real food. Scientists have been able to produce foods that do not satiate and increase your hunger for more. Ever heard of the Lays potato chip slogan of "betcha can't eat just one?" The colors and flavors found in our food today are not at all what is found in nature. It is man-made. It's made just for you. We need Nancy Reagan again, reminding us what she taught us when I was 9 years old, "Just Say No."

In order to sell you garbage and label it as food, it takes more than clever ingredients and package marketing to convince you. Food companies have become like the Great and Powerful Oz. They don't want us to see what is behind that curtain. In order to make us feel better about what we eat, they are going as far as masking the names of certain ingredients in order to trick you, and even lying about the ingredients, making false claims! Most people probably don't know that words like high fructose corn syrup, maltodextrin, dextrose, sucrose, barley malt syrup, and maltose are all the same as SUGAR! Or how about the "no sugar added" claim? Could you imagine if they added even more sugar to the already sugar laced packs of goodies? It doesn't mean that is it sugar-free. It's a marketing ploy to make you feel better.

So, it begs the question, how then, do we even begin to eat with quality in mind? It can seem daunting and impractical, especially after what you have just read. The food manufacturers are out to get you and there is no escape, right? Wrong. It may not be easy, but it is possible. I have developed my personal training business so that I am taking my clients to the supermarket as well as the gym. I have spent hours with folks walking around their favorite grocery, helping them to see how to circumnavigate the store to stay out of the "danger" sections. Usually the outer perimeter is the safest and freshest food areas. Then, we spend time learning food labels. I teach them how to read the false claims and marketing gimmicks on the front of the packages, as well as the ingredient lists and the nutrient lists. Education is vital. You must educate yourself on what you are being sold.

Now, set some standards. I believe God wants us to eat food the way He created it. Prepared, not processed. This can be difficult, but we can make steps in the right direction and reap some amazing results. How do we do this? Try to eat food that you can name all or at least most of the ingredients in it. If you eat an apple, guess what? There is one ingredient. Apple. If you eat packaged apple chips, you are consuming an apple, plus additives that you do not know what they are. And probably added sugar. If you eat chicken, then eat fresh, or at least canned chicken. Not processed chicken served frozen in a box. One of my favorite meals to prepare is a relatively quick and super easy meal: pan fried wild caught Sockeye salmon in coconut oil, steamed broccoli with cheese and grass-fed butter, and a sweet potato. All with a dash of sea salt. Mmmgood! Not only did I just list my favorite meal, but I also listed every ingredient in the meal!

Pay the money. Too often people complain about the prices of whole food. I get it. Times are hard and money is short. If you're feeding a family like me, it is a problem that is only compounded. I believe this is a matter of perspective. Here's what I mean. It's not necessarily that whole food is expensive…it's that processed food is so cheap! Cheap quality gets a cheap price tag. One day my sons and I ventured into our local market where we like to buy bulk items. This saves money. I needed nuts. And so, to the bulk nut and seed isle we go. There is also bulk candy in this isle. My raw almonds were $9 per pound. The jellybeans that my youngest protested for were less than $1 per pound. Nine dollars for real nutrient dense food, or a couple of bucks for wasted health damaging garbage? Would you pay nine dollars to add healthful benefits to your body, or would you pay a few bucks to add sickness and disease to your body? To me, it's a no-brainer. But, consider this: that in this life, you are going to pay for healthcare. You can either put your money in the front end of your health through eating a high-quality diet and preventing disease, or, you can put your money on the back end of your life, using it for medications, doctors, hospital bills, and so on. Both are expensive. The former will provide quality and quantity of life. The latter will hardly provide either. So, think of your food as preventative medicine. As the great Greek philosopher Hippocrates once said, "Let food be thy medicine and medicine be thy food."

I could write a volume of books on how to eat, giving insight to genetic markers, bio-individuality, blood type, gut microbiome, and so forth. All of which, and more, are important to finding out the best foods for a person to eat. We will save for another day, discussions on diet plans and specific eating regimens; vegetarian, carnivore, vegan, low-carb, keto, etc. etc. I want to leave you with some very simple yet practical principles for approaching your plate with high quality. Here's my list.

1. Do not consume processed sugar.
2. Stay away from plant oils such as canola, soy, corn, cottonseed, sunflower or peanut oil. Instead use healthy animal fats (butter, ghee, lard) as well as coconut, avocado, and extra virgin olive oil.
3. Purchase pasture raised, grass-fed beef and butter.
4. Get cage-free, omnivore (not grain-fed) chickens and eggs.
5. Choose wild caught fish.
6. Opt for fresh or frozen vegetables
7. Do not use artificial sweeteners (allulose, sucralose, etc.). Stevia is not artificial, so it is allowable.
8. Be able to name all or most of all the ingredients in your food.
9. Limit the handling of your food to 3 people. A great way to do this is to shop farmers markets.
10. Stay away from Genetically Modified Organisms (GMOs) and pesticides.

Even if we're to just start here with this list, you would immediately reap the benefits of better health. Approaching our plate with quality control does much to honor our body. I believe it is God's will for us to think this way. The Apostle John opens his 3rd letter to his friend and co-ministry leader, Gaius, by saying,

"The Elder: To my dear friend Gaius: I love you in the truth. Dear friend, I pray that you may prosper in every way and be in good health physically just as you are spiritually." (verses 1-3)

It is good to nurture our physical body with whole, fresh food. But, it's not just for us. In doing so, we honor the Lord as well. We are receiving and accepting what He has given us, without altering it. We are seeing it for the true beauty and gift that it is, in its natural state. We are essentially saying, "It is good and doesn't need to be improved." That honors God. And, so does our attention to nurturing our bodies in order to carry out His work.

With Purpose

Why do you eat? Well, we have already covered why you were created to eat. But, why do you eat the way you eat? What is the purpose behind your diet? Ask anyone. After the awkward moment of confusion, answers will begin to stream. The first being that they are hungry. This is an easy, and obvious answer. It's called innate intelligence. Our body produces a hormone called Leptin, which sends a signal to the brain activating the hunger signals. These signals then send messages to the gut, where it begins to produce acids that will be used to break down foods. You are aware of this sequence when your tummy begins to growl at you. This is what we call hunger. Another answer is a little more goal oriented. Some may answer with 'weight loss/fat loss.' Perhaps the reason you eat the way you do is to lose some unwanted fat stores. When we decrease insulin (the fat storing hormone) by decreasing glucose, our body begins to look for another fuel source. It remembers the fat that it stored on your frame and begins to mobilize it for energy use. Or, if you are in a calorie deficit, you will also trigger the body's desire for energy and see a reduction in fat. It doesn't take much to notice that this is a popular reason people eat the way they do. Oddly, or ironically enough, we are reminded of the latest and greatest diet for getting into that summer ready body, while we are checking out at the grocery. All the magazines in the checkout isle are giving us the latest scoop. Some who are willing to be honest enough might admit they eat because they love to eat. Food tastes good and they love eating good tasting food. They see what looks, smells or tastes good and they go for it. I've had lots of people tell me they are on a "see" food diet. They eat the food they see.

I'd like to offer another purpose: the Gospel.

Because I lend so much support and attention to my own diet, I have been labeled a "health nut." I've been called this by fellow believers. For some reason, in the church, we have gotten the idea that God is only interested in our spiritual health. We cling to:

"For the training of the body has a limited benefit, but godliness is beneficial in every way, since it holds promise for the present life and also for the life to come." 1 Timothy 4:8

We use this verse to discredit physical fitness and proper eating instead of elevating it. By using comparison and contrasting, we justify paying little to no attention to the physical body. Though I believe it to be rationalization by guilt. We use this verse, making a true statement, but for the cause of thwarting pour responsibility. Training of the body does have only limited benefit. Of course. Flesh and blood in and of itself is limited; limited in strength, limited by time, limited by the curse of sin. One day it will perish, regardless of what you do. There is nothing more beneficial than godliness in our lives. To love and obey our Lord is of the utmost importance. Amen. That is not to say that the training of the body is without benefit that we should be concerned.

While wandering the wilderness for 40 years, God dwelt among His people in a temporary tent made of skin, called the Tabernacle. This shelter was designed by God, Himself. Every inch, every piece of material, was given by instruction from the Lord for the people, the artisans, builders, and craftsman to build. God put enormous detail into a structure that would house His glory.

Afterwards, God allowed Solomon to build a monumental structure on the holiest of mountains in Jerusalem. This building would rival any and all other buildings in beauty and purpose. King Solomon's Temple, if left standing today, would be considered the eighth wonder of the world. Solomon spared no expense. He brought great cedars from Lebanon. Gold and granite from miles away. This Temple was to the glory of God; a place where He would dwell in the Holy of Holies.

The tabernacle was replaced by the Temple. In 587 BC, the Babylonians with their king Nebuchadnezzar, destroyed the Temple. This left the Jews disgraced for many years, and eventually they all but forgot about it. Until the Prophet Haggai:

"The word of the Lord came through Haggai the prophet: 'Is it a time for you yourselves to live in your paneled houses, while this house lies in ruins?' Now, the Lord of Hosts says this: Think carefully about your ways. You have planted much but harvested little. You eat but never have enough to be satisfied. You drink but never have enough to become drunk. You put on clothes but never have enough to get warm. The wage earner puts his wages into a bag with a hole in it. 'The Lord of Hosts says this: Think carefully about your ways. Go up into the hills, bring down lumber, and build the house. Then I will be pleased with it and be glorified,' says the Lord." Haggai 1:4-8

It was a disgrace to leave the house of God broken down. Though it was merely a building made of stone, its purpose was divine.

After the rebuilding of the Temple came subsequent celebrations, commemorations, and use for many years. In the year AD 70, the Romans, under the direction of Nero burned Jerusalem to the ground, destroying once again God's holy temple. One day, we know that this temple will once again be rebuilt and will usher in a new season of glorification. Until then, there is another temple that needs to be rebuilt.

"Don't you know that your body is a sanctuary of the Holy Spirit who is in you, whom you have from God? You are not your own, for you were bought at a price. Therefore glorify God in your body."
1 Corinthians 6:19-20

When Christ died upon the cross, and the veil of the Temple was torn into, He was changing once again the Temple location. The veil that separated the Holy of Holies, where the presence of God dwelt, from all people was now obsolete. It wasn't so that we could enter that sacred room and the presence of God, but so that God could enter into each of us, making us sacred unto Himself. As we submit and give our lives to trust in and follow Jesus Christ, God the father sets up residence in us through the presence of His Holy Spirit. My friend, you are the temple of God.

Your body was specifically designed by our Creator. Design was laid out in detail to cover every micro character and purpose of who you are.

"I will praise You because I have been remarkably and wonderfully made. Your works are wonderful, and I know this very well. My bones were not hidden from You when I was made in secret, when I was formed in the depths of the earth. Your eyes saw me when I was formless; all my days were written in Your book and planned before a single one of them began."
Psalms 139:14-16

Though your body is made of perishable material, it is the temple of the Most Holy, and is to be used to glorify Him in both activity and health.

"Don't you know that your body is a sanctuary of the Holy Spirit who is in you, whom you have from God? You are not your own, for you were bought at a price. Therefore glorify God in your body."
1 Corinthians 6:19, 20

Like the prophet Haggai, I believe there is a mandate of God calling out to His children to "rebuild the house." His people are broken down and disgraced. We are not the healthiest people on the planet, but shouldn't we be? What is our testimony before the world as followers of a Book that commands glorification in our bodies?

We can and should glorify God in two ways with our bodies. First, let's steward it well by honoring him in it. Our actions in this physical frame should always glorify God. Sin may start in the mind, but it is carried out in the flesh. We have already talked about gluttony and drunkenness. Have you ever considered, however, how God views the food that we eat and the damage that it does? He provided wonderful, nutritious food to develop and build our bodies. We can't blame the Babylonians and Romans for the destruction of this temple. This time, the destroyers are us! We are consuming food that tears down the body. By what we eat, we are creating inflammation and oxidized stress that leads to disease and death. By what we eat, we are destroying our health and the ability to serve God and carry out His will in our lives.

God's calling on your life probably necessitates having a physical body to carry it out. Am I right? What if you don't have enough energy? What if you are not physically able? Better yet, let me give you a scenario.

Meet Brother Bill. He's pastor of a large and thriving church. There are lots of responsibilities for Bro. Bill to see to. He often visits the sick, elderly, and those in the hospital. He is on the road often, making meetings and working with community leaders. He spends ample time studying and preparing for his Sunday and min-week teachings. Bro. Bill is the husband to Dorothy and father to their 3 teenage children.

Bro. Bill doesn't pay attention to his diet. He has too little time for that. He eats fast food while on the road. No time for breakfast. Last year was his 45th birthday. Mornings are getting harder to get up and get going. So is his sex life. He just can't seem to feel as romantic as he once could. The desire is there, but he just can't seem to perform. He's ashamed and embarrassed and doesn't want to talk about it. Dorothy thinks it's her fault and that she is no longer attractive to him. She battles depression now. Bill doesn't have the energy to play and rough house with his kids these days. His body is tight, and he feels aches and pains that weren't there last year.

Bro. Bill's decrease of energy and mental lethargy is causing a lack of performance in the church as well. The deacons have noticed and reprimand him. People are starting to notice the tired wrinkles under his eyes and begin to talk. He is stressed.

Dorothy and Bro. Bill fight a lot now. Their marriage is on the rocks and she's considered leaving. Bill, tired, broken, and embarrassed, is considering leaving the ministry altogether.

Bro. Bill's story isn't uncommon. But Bro. Bill's story is not entirely explained. Bill reached an age that his testosterone (the male sex hormone) naturally falls and dips low. This is normal but preventable. This would explain his lost sex drive. Bro. Bill has accumulated oxidized stress in his body from consuming highly inflammatory, rancid fast food vegetable oils for years. Both his wife and his children suffer for it. The emotional and physical stress put a toll on Bills adrenal glands, causing them to secrete higher amounts of the stress hormone cortisol. These elevated levels cause Bro. Bill to feel tired and moody, constantly.

It's not the end of the road for Bro. Bill, but it will be a long road back to restore his health, his marriage, and his church because he did not glorify God in his body. His neglect of the sanctuary of God prevented him from being who and what God had called him to be. It wasn't for a lack of desire. Perhaps Bro. Bill just brushed it off as "the training of the body is limited benefit."

This doesn't have to be the case.

By glorifying God in our body, we can then glorify God with our body. By eating the right foods, getting the proper rest, exercising adequately, and supplementing smart, we can do more than prevent the breakdown that leads to handicapping our calling; we can optimize it!

We are 100% spirit. That's 'who' we are. But your spirit is not free from your body! You HAVE to have that physical transport in shape to carry you around and do the things you've been called to do. I want to shout this from the roof tops. Your life while on this planet will always be both physical and spiritual. To separate the two is called death. So, let's stop separating them. When you feel bad physically, it causes low feelings emotionally. When you are not in a good emotional place, it can and will cause problems in your body. Chronic stress wreaks havoc on the body.

"If you take care of your body and your brain, you are that much better able to defend the Gospel, to make a defense for the hope that is with you; and so, having a combination of physical culture and mental culture, combined with Christianity is potent and powerful combination." - Ben Greenfield [2]

Our purpose is the Gospel. If we are going to put as much attention into our spiritual lives to be transformed by it, shouldn't we treat our bodies so they are able to carry it out? Honoring God in it by what we eat will allow for us to honor God with it, to carry out the message of the Gospel in word, and in deed.

One of my heroes from old is Caleb in the Old Testament. As a young man, he was sent by Moses to go with Joshua and ten others to spy out the land promised by God for Israelites to inhabit. Fear overtook ten of the spies as they saw giant men in fortified cities. Because of their false narrative, God did not allow that generation to inherit the land. By the time a new generation had come along, and Caleb, now in his eighties, God leads them in. Caleb reminds the Israelites what was given to him as a young man, believing that is still God's calling upon his life.

"As you see, the Lord has kept me alive these 45 years as He promised, since the Lord spoke this word to Moses while Israel was journeying in the wilderness. Here I am today, 85 years old. I am still as strong today as I was the day Moses sent me out. My strength for battle and for daily tasks is now as it was then. Now give me this hill country the Lord promised me on that day, because you heard then that the Anakim are there, as well as large fortified cities." Joshua 14:10-12

Oh, if that could be said of all of us. I desire to serve my King in old age as well, if not better than I did as a young man. Every meal that I ingest and every bite I swallow is either working for that purpose or against it. If you were to ask me why I eat the way that I do, my answer is simple: the Gospel.

As a pharmacy

How much does the average American spend on non-preventable medication a year? In 2016, we spent $329 BILLION dollars on pharmaceutical medicine! That's billion with a "b." [3]

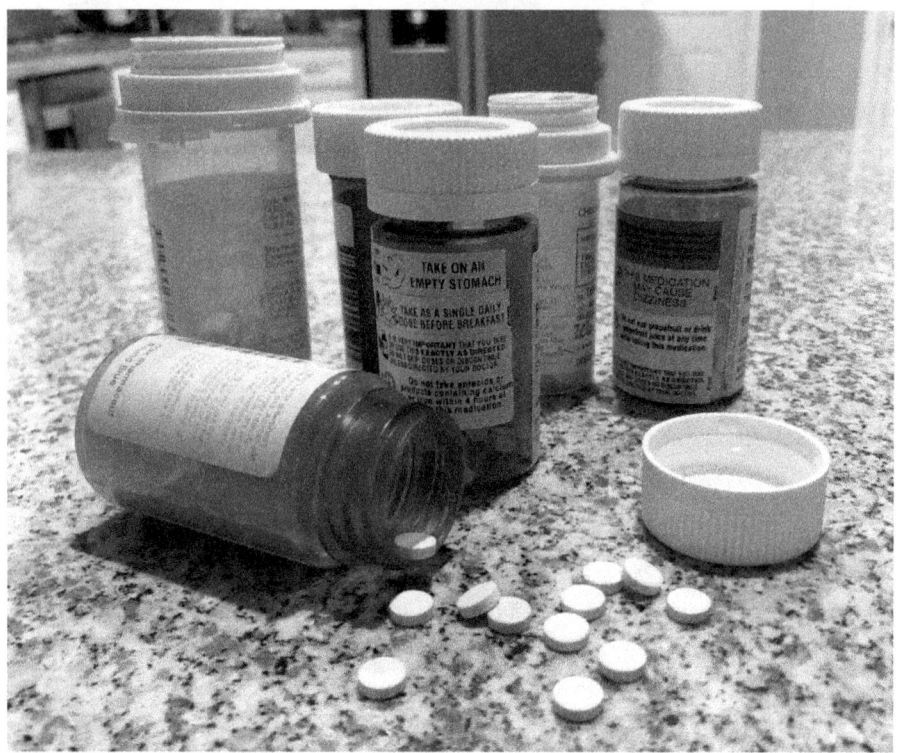

Medications are prescribed abundantly throughout the United States every day. Just go into any pharmacy and you can see how busy they are as they fill prescriptions as fast as they can. Here's a list of the top ten prescribed drugs in the U.S. How many of these do are you taking?

According to MedicineNet, the top 10 drugs prescribed to Americans in 2018 were:

1. Vicodin (hydrocodone/acetaminophen)

Vicodin is a popular drug for treating acute or chronic moderate to moderately severe pain. Its most common side effects are lightheadedness, dizziness, sedation, nausea, and vomiting. Vicodin can reduce breathing, impair thinking, reduce physical abilities, and is habit forming.

2. Simvastatin (Generic for Zocor)

Simvastatin is one of the first "statins" (HMG-CoA reductase inhibitors) approved for treating high cholesterol and reducing the risk of stroke, death from heart disease, and risk of heart attacks. Its most common side effects are headache, nausea, vomiting, diarrhea, abdominal pain, and muscle pain. Like other statins it can cause muscle break down.

3. Lisinopril (Generic for Prinivil or Zestril)

Lisinopril is an angiotensin converting enzyme (ACE) inhibitor used for treating high blood pressure, congestive heart failure, and for preventing kidney failure caused by high blood pressure and diabetes. Lisinopril side effects include dizziness, nausea, headaches, drowsiness, and sexual dysfunction. ACE inhibitors may cause a dry cough that resolves when the drug is discontinued.

4. Levothyroxine (generic for Synthroid)

Levothryoxine is a man-made version of thyroid hormone. It is used for treating hypothyroidism. Its side effects are usually result from high levels of thyroid hormone. Excessive thyroid hormone can cause chest pain, increased heart rate, excessive sweating, heat intolerance, nervousness, headache, and weight loss.

5. Azithromycin (generic for Zithromax, Z-PAK)

Azithromycin is an antibiotic used for treating ear, throat, and sinus infections as well as pneumonia, bronchitis, and some sexually transmitted diseases. Its common side effects include loose stools, nausea, stomach pain, and vomiting. Rare side effects include abnormal liver tests, allergic reactions, nervousness, and abnormal heart beats.

6. Metformin (generic for Glucophage)

Metformin is used alone or in combination with other drugs for treating type 2 diabetes in adults and children. The most common side effects of metformin are nausea, vomiting, gas, bloating, diarrhea, and loss of appetite.

7. Lipitor (atorvastatin)

Lipitor is a "statin" (HMG-CoA reductase inhibitors) approved for treating high cholesterol. It also prevents chest pain, stroke, heart attack in individuals with coronary artery disease. It causes minor side effects such as constipation, diarrhea, fatigue, gas, heartburn, and headache. Like other statins it can cause muscle pain and muscle break down.

8. Amlodipine (generic for Norvasc)

Amlodipine is a calcium channel blocker used for treating high blood pressure and for treatment and prevention of chest pain. Its most common side effects are headache and swelling of the lower extremities. Amlodipine can also cause dizziness, flushing, fatigue, nausea, and palpitations.

9. Amoxicillin

Amoxicillin is a penicillin type antibiotic used for treating several types of bacterial infections such as ear, tonsils, throat, larynx, urinary tract, and skin infections. Its side effects are diarrhea, heartburn, nausea, itching, vomiting, confusion, abdominal pain, rash, and allergic reactions.

10. Hydrochlorothiazide

Hydrochlorothiazide is a diuretic (water pill) used alone or combined with other drugs for treating high blood pressure. Its side effects include weakness, low blood pressure, light sensitivity, impotence, nausea, abdominal pain, electrolyte disturbances, and rash. [4]

I lament this list. I believe we are spending billions of hard-earned dollars on medications or illnesses that are either completely preventable, and/or unnecessary as a treatment. I am not saying that they don't work. I'm just saying that if we approach food the way it is intended, we would subsequently abolish the reasons for having to take these medications; we could either prevent the illness or cure it.

The Greek philosopher Hippocrates is noted for saying, "Let food be thy medicine, and medicine be thy food." I ascribe to such a philosophy.

When is the last time you found yourself standing in line at your local pharmacy? I am eternally grateful for my doctor and my pharmacist, but I loathe the process of prescription care: the time spent in a cold waiting room, followed by more time spent in a cold exam room that could have been better spent doing something that I actually enjoy! The last time I went to the pharmacy, I learned that my script was late. I had to wait around for over an hour just to pick it up. When I finally got it, the cost at check-out was enough to give me heart attack! Then, we fill our medicine cabinets with all the pills that we have to remember to take on a daily basis. By the way, has it ever occurred to anyone that it is absurd that we have an entire cabinet devoted to 'medicine'? And if that isn't enough, for every pharmaceutical that sits in our cabinet, is a list of side effects that makes the illness in which we are fighting pale in comparison to the risk of taking the medication! I remember a commercial for a popular anti-depressant that came with a possible side-effect of suicide. The same side-effect could be found with a popular smoking cessation drug. So, if the depression and the cigarettes don't kill you, the drug just might! One popular weight loss drug warns of "anal seepage." This drug should work. I can't imagine even wanting to eat knowing that risk! Weight loss should be a piece of cake…pun intended.

We have become a drug induced society. Our current lifestyles create diseased states that require medical attention. With every symptom, we demand a quick fix. And we are willing to face the risks and pay the money.

What if we approached food as a pharmacy? We might do that if we understand that that is a huge part of the intent of food. We might do that if we understand the design of the human body is created with the ability to fight, prevent, and cure illness and disease, but that it requires the right food to do so. We might if we saw that as a cheaper, easier, and more successful route than that of modern pharma.

You have another medicine cabinet in your home. As a matter of fact, you have an entire room devoted to medicine. It's called a kitchen. That doesn't mean you actually have medicine stored there though. The typical westerner has more stored poisons and toxins in their kitchen than actual medicine. Nevertheless, it could and should be stocked full of medicine called real food.

When we look at food as medicine, we start to see what makes it medicine--nutrients. God has created within all substance meant for consumption, nutrients. A nutrient is a substance that provides nourishment essential for growth and the maintenance of life. It's used by an organism to survive, grow, and reproduce. The requirement for dietary nutrient intake applies to animals, plants, fungi, and protists. You cannot survive without them. Oddly enough, we are at the same time obese and malnourished. Due to consuming more nutrient lacking calories, we find a state of health that is paradoxical.

Food that is dense in nutrients contains the building blocks for health: vitamins, minerals, fats, proteins, enzymes, etc.

Micro-Nutrients

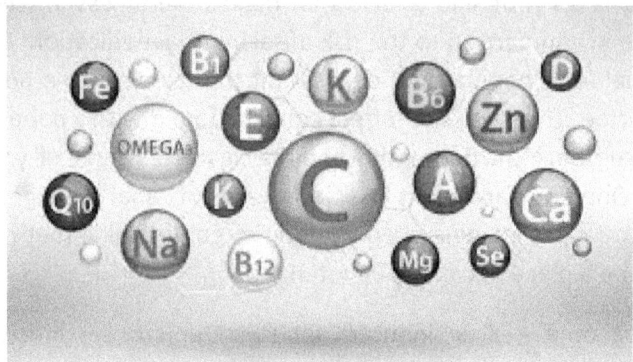

Micro-nutrients are vital for human health. These tiny nutrients are vitamins and minerals. The 13 essential vitamins your body needs are vitamins A, C, D, E, K and the B vitamins: thiamine (B1), riboflavin (B2), niacin (B3), pantothenic acid (B5), pyroxidine (B6), biotin (B7), folate (B9) and cobalamin (B12). The four fat-soluble vitamins—A, D, E, and K—are stored in the body's fatty tissues.

Vitamins play many important roles in your body, such as maintaining healthy eyes and skin, acting as antioxidants to protect your cells from damage, and contributing to healthy reproduction and growth, strong bones and normal blood clotting. Different vitamins are found in foods from grains, vegetables, fruits, dairy products, and meats/beans. There are 16 essential minerals: calcium, phosphorus, potassium, sulfur, sodium, chloride, magnesium, iron, zinc, copper, manganese, iodine, and selenium, molybdenum, chromium, and fluoride. Minerals play important roles in maintaining blood pressure, fluid & electrolyte balance, and bone health, making new cells, delivering oxygen to cells, and contributing to normal muscle and nerve functioning.

You can go to a pharmacy or supplement shop and stock up on bottles of supplements to get all of these micronutrients, or... you can get them all from eating real food.

Micronutrients do not provide energy. Meaning, they do not contain calories. But they are responsible for the release of energy from macronutrients. Macronutrients are listed as protein, carbohydrate, and fat. Everything you eat will be classified as one of these 3 or a mixture of the three.

Protein

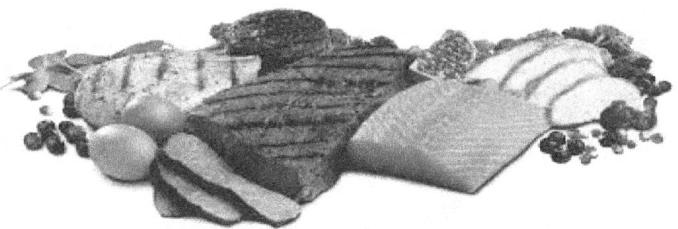

Protein is found in meat sources primarily. All meat is protein. You can also find protein in some vegetables and milk. Protein, after digestion, gets broken down into amino acids. Amino acids are the structural building blocks of the body. All skin, muscle, bone, hair, teeth, etc., is made up of amino acids. Amino acids are essential to life, and so you must eat protein.

Carbohydrates

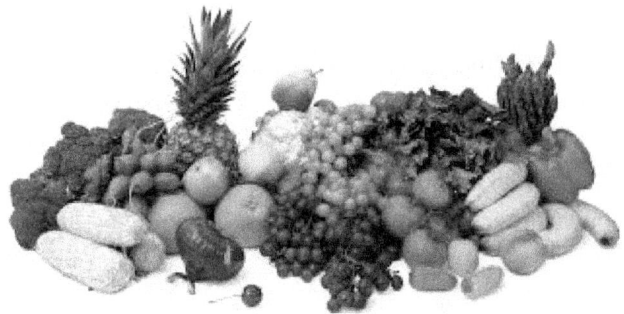

Carbohydrates are found in vegetables, fruits, grains, and sugars. Though there is no such thing as an "essential" carbohydrate, they serve a very important role in the body. When a carbohydrate is digested, it is broken down into forms of sugar in the body, either glucose or fructose. Once introduced in the blood, it causes a hormone effect that raises insulin which will shuttle the sugars into the cells for energy. Carbs can be divided into two classifications based on the ability to be broken down quickly or slowly: simple and complex. Simple carbs break down quick and are used quick, causing "spikes" in blood sugar levels. Complex carbs are slowly digested, thereby causing a slower release of insulin and longer sustained levels of blood sugar. An example of simple carbs would be sugar, pasta, honey, and fruit. An example of complex carbs would be oats, fibrous vegetables, and whole grains.

Fat

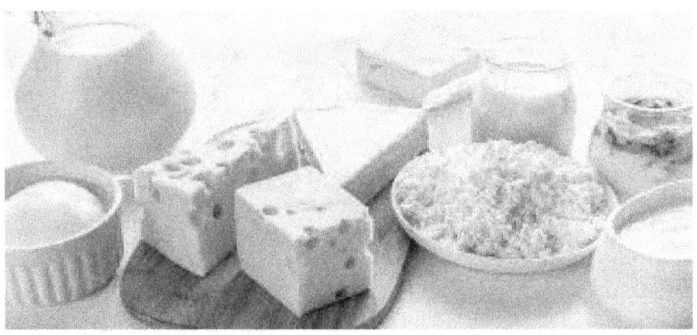

Fat is another essential nutrient. Fat is found in things like olive oil, coconut oil, avocado oil, butter and ghee. It is also found in foods such as eggs, nuts, and cheeses. Fat enters the body and is broken down into fatty acids and glycerol. These fatty acids play a major role in the body's production, transport, and modulation of hormones and cholesterol. There is a huge difference between "good fats" and "bad fats" that needs to be stated. Bad fats such as hydrogenated cooking oils and fake butters are man-made, toxic killers. These fats cause inflammation and oxidation in the body that lead to a myriad of diseases. Good fats are natural and healthy, and despite marketing, do not make you fat. Good fat gives you energy, satiates your hunger, and builds important hormones vital for optimal health.

Water

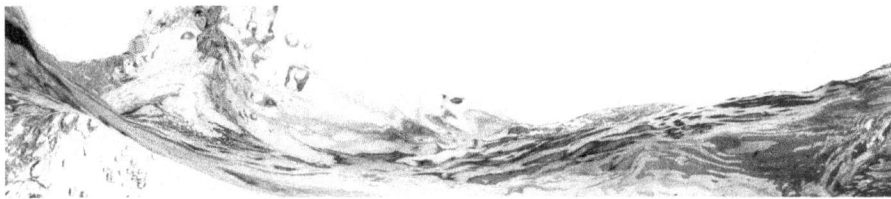

Though water is not a "nutrient" by definition, it is obviously essential for sustaining life. I recommend drinking about 2 liters of water daily. Even when we are slightly dehydrated, we can suffer headaches, hunger pains, mental fatigue, and lethargy.

All these nutrients that I have mentioned are found in food sources. Only when we are not able to get adequate levels from food, should we use supplementation. But here's the thing. Your body was uniquely created to use all of these nutrients in order to produce and sustain optimal health. It's like a combination lock. When you combine the right nutrients in the right amounts, your body unlocks its potential to prevent and fight illness and heal itself. Your body, as "fearfully and wonderfully" made, is specifically designed for this. Every second of your life, there is at work, processes taking place- enzymatic, hormonal, genetic, bacterial, neuronal, electrical-all these processes that you never think about. Why? Because it is innate intelligence at work. God has created your body to function autonomically to survive. But there's a caveat; you have to give it what it needs.

For instance, running throughout your entire body are blood vessels. From the largest arteries to the smallest capillaries, your blood vessels transport fluids that contain the vitamins, minerals, and nutrients that have been designed to fuel and build your body. Lining every square inch of your capillaries are tiny little cells called endothelium. These endothelial cells are like tiny little medicine bottles. I'm over-simplifying of course but hang with me. Imagine your entire body has running through it its own pharmacy. These endothelial cells are the medicine bottles waiting to dispense the necessary medicine to boost your immune system and heal your body. Approach food so that you see it this way. Real food opens the lids of these bottles. Real food contains the nutrients that opens them up. Processed food and junk food do the opposite. Unhealthy food causes inflammation and oxidation that prevents these medicine bottles from opening. Imagine a sticky sludge that has glued the lids shut.

Many people will spend large amounts of money and time, and insurance premiums in order to treat chronic, preventable illnesses, and complain that they cannot afford to eat whole, real food. My argument is, you are going to pay for healthcare regardless. Your choice is, at which end of your life you will pay for it. You can spend the money up front and eat food that will stave off illness or spend it at the end of your life to treat illness. I choose to spend the extra money on quality medicine that I enjoy taking and that tastes great, rather than the latter.

The best medicine money can buy. Isn't that what we all want, ideally? But does that come in a pill? Of course not! God has provided us with the absolute best medicine, and He did it from the very beginning of creation. What He has provided was not just to be enjoyed for taste or satiation. It's the good, delicious taste that makes the medicine go down. He has wrapped all of nature's good healing power inside of mouth-watering goodness. As the old saying goes, "an apple a day keeps the doctor away." Well, it may take more than just an apple, but nevertheless, what He has provided can indeed keep the doctor away, at least much more so than commonly practiced. And so, what is the best medicine money can buy? I believe it is fresh, whole, real food. Organic and unaltered. I'm not prescribing a diet. I'm simply saying that the best food medicine is the best food, and the best food is intact and unadulterated by man's processing. Here are my rules of thumb:

Rule #1.

Find the best meats. Wild game is by far the best meat. Deer, elk, antelope, rabbit, etc. These animals are free range, grass fed, hormone free perfection. And, the best, most nutritious part of these animals, their organs. That's right. Heart, kidney, liver, brain, spleen. These are the most nutrient dense part of the animals. The Native Americans prized these organ meats far above the skeletal muscle of the animal. [When I was a boy, growing up in the country and woodlands, hunting was a normal part of life. We were friends and neighbors with a family that would help us process our game. I can remember the old grandmother, Bessy Mae, who came out to inspect our work. She would rummage through the discarded animal parts, shaking her head at our refusal of the organs. She would load up her hands with deer heart and brains, and head back into the house satisfied that she had obtained the best part of the animal.] If you can't obtain wild game where you live, try not to settle for anything less than grass-fed, hormone free, and free ranged beef and bison. Wild caught sockeye salmon. Free-range, cage free chickens and eggs. Butter from the same grass-fed stock at the beef.

Rule #2.

Purchase the best vegetables. I recommend supporting your local farmer's market. There, you will often find fruits and vegetables that are locally grown, without pesticides and GMOs. I love vegetables and I try to get as many colors as possible. I also try to get as nutrient dense vegetables as I can. Many of those can be found in leafy greens and cruciferous vegetables, such a kale, chard, broccoli, Brussels sprouts, bok choy, asparagus, and cauliflower.

Rule #3.

Consume the best fats. Remember that synthetically made, hydrogenated fats have adverse effects on our health. These rancid oils such a canola, vegetable oil, palm oil, and margarine are high in Omega-6 fatty acids and lead to an increase in arterial, joint, and brain inflammation and oxidation. The best oils are those God has given to us. Grass-fed butter and ghee, cold pressed olive oil, unrefined coconut oil, and avocado oil are some of the best oils and fats on the planet.

Rule #4.

Stick with the best grains. Honestly, I limit my consumption of grains to a minimum altogether. Chronically high levels of insulin are damaging to the body, and too much fiber is inflaming to the gut. Occasionally I do enjoy some grains, and I am very particular to which grains I choose. I stay away from bleached, enriched white flour. My first and favorite go-to grain for health would be sour dough. This fermented grain is easier on the gut and acts as a probiotic, feeding the gut bacteria. After that, I search for things like rye, barley, oat, and millet.

Herbs

Another food that is worth mentioning as a medicine is herbs. Herbs are plants that are specifically used to treat ailments and illnesses. They may come from leaves, roots, seeds, bark, or the fruit of a plant. Cinnamon has been touted as a great way to lower post-prandial blood sugar. White willow bark has been used for centuries for headaches.

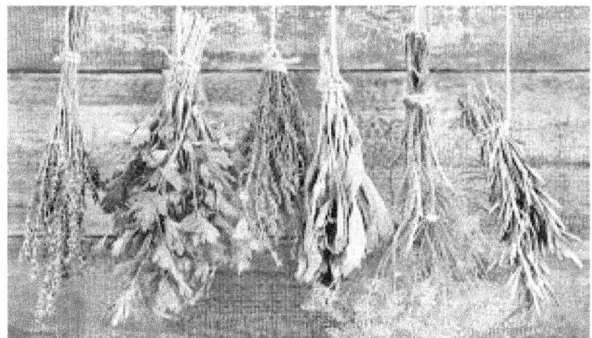

Here is a list compiled by the University of Rochester Medical Center that explains some common herbs and their influence of health.

Chamomile

Considered by some to be a cure-all, chamomile is commonly used in the U.S. as anxiolytic and sedative for anxiety and relaxation. It is used in Europe for wound healing and to reduce inflammation or swelling. Few studies have looked at how well it works for any condition. Chamomile is used as a tea or applied as a compress. It is considered safe by the FDA. It may increase drowsiness caused by medicines or other herbs or supplements. Chamomile may interfere with the way the body uses some medicines, causing too high a level of the medicine in some people. As with any medicinal herb, talk with your healthcare provider before taking it.

Echinacea

Echinacea is commonly used to treat or prevent colds, flu, and infections, and for wound healing. More than 25 published studies looked at how well Echinacea worked to prevent or shorten the course of a cold, but none were conclusive. A 2014 study compared Echinacea with a placebo for treating colds. Results found that Echinacea did not have any effect on a cold. Other studies have also shown that long-term use can affect the body's immune system. It should not be used with medicines that can cause liver problems. People allergic to plants in the daisy family may be more likely to have an allergic reaction to Echinacea. The daisy family includes ragweed, chrysanthemums, marigolds, and daisies.

Feverfew

Feverfew was traditionally used to treat fevers. It is now commonly used to prevent migraines and treat arthritis. Some research has shown that certain feverfew preparations can prevent migraines. Side effects include mouth ulcers and digestive irritation. People who suddenly stop taking feverfew for migraines may have their headaches return. Feverfew should not be used with nonsteroidal anti-inflammatory medicines because these medicines may change how well feverfew works. It should not be used with warfarin or other anticoagulant medicines.

Garlic

Garlic is used for lowering cholesterol and blood pressure. It has antimicrobial effects. Reports from small, short-term, and poorly described studies show that it may cause small reductions in total and LDL cholesterol. But German research results on garlic's cholesterol-lowering effect have been distorted for a positive effect, the FDA says. Researchers are currently exploring garlic's possible role in preventing cancer. The FDA considers garlic safe. It should not be used with warfarin, because large amounts of garlic may affect clotting. For the same reason, large amounts should not be taken before dental procedures or surgery.

Ginger

Ginger is used to ease nausea and motion sickness. Research suggests that ginger can relieve nausea caused by pregnancy or chemotherapy. Other areas under investigation are in surgery and for nausea caused by motion.

Gingko

Ginkgo leaf extract has been used to treat a variety of conditions such as asthma, bronchitis, fatigue, and tinnitus. It is also used to improve memory and to prevent dementia and other brain disorders. Only extract from leaves should be used. Seeds contain ginkgo toxin. This toxin can cause seizures and, in large amounts, death. Because some information suggests that ginkgo can increase the risk of bleeding, it should not be used with nonsteroidal anti-inflammatory medicines, anticoagulants, anticonvulsant medicines, or tricyclic antidepressants.

Ginseng

Ginseng is used as a tonic and aphrodisiac, even as a cure-all. Research is uncertain how well it works, partly because of the difficulty in defining "vitality" and "quality of life." There is a large variation in the quality of ginseng sold. Side effects are high blood pressure and tachycardia. It's considered safe by the FDA, but shouldn't be used with warfarin, heparin, nonsteroidal anti-inflammatory medicines, estrogens, corticosteroids, or digoxin. People with diabetes should not use ginseng.

Goldenseal

Goldenseal is used to treat diarrhea, and eye and skin irritations. It is also used as an antiseptic. It is also an unproven treatment for colds. Goldenseal contains berberine, a plant alkaloid with a long history of medicinal use in both Ayurvedic and Chinese medicine. Studies have shown that goldenseal is effective for diarrhea. But it's not recommended because it can be poisonous in high doses. It can cause skin, mouth, throat, and gastric irritation. It is also not recommended because of the plant's endangered species status.

Milk Thistle

Milk thistle is used to treat liver conditions and high cholesterol, and to reduce the growth of cancer cells. Milk thistle is a plant that originated in the Mediterranean region. It has been used for many different illnesses over the last several thousand years, especially liver problems. Although study results are uncertain, some promising information exists.

Passion Flower

Passion Flower makes a tea that promotes sleep and anti-anxiety. The flower, leaves and stem are all used for making Passion Flower tea.

Saint John's Wort

Saint John's wort is used as an antidepressant. Recent studies have not confirmed that there is more than a slight effect on depression. More research is needed to determine the best dose. A side effect is sensitivity to light, but this is only noted in people taking large doses of the herb. St. John's work can cause a dangerous interaction with other commonly used medicines. Always talk with your healthcare provider before using this herb.

Valerian

Valerian is used to treat sleeplessness and to reduce anxiety. Research suggests that valerian may be a helpful sleep aid, but there are no well-designed studies to confirm the results. In the U.S., valerian is used as a flavoring for root beer and other foods. As with any medicinal herb, talk with your healthcare provider before taking it. [5]

I have taken herbs my entire life as a means of medicinal health. I find comfort from Scripture that this is God's intended use for herbs. In a prophetic vision of the restored Kingdom, Ezekiel records:

"All kinds of trees providing food will grow along both banks of the river. Their leaves will not wither, and their fruit will not fail. Each month they will bear fresh fruit because the water comes from the sanctuary. Their fruit will be used for food and their leaves for medicine." Ezekiel 47:12

And we will see again, as John the Revelator sheds light on our forever home in the new kingdom:

"...The tree of life was on both sides of the river, bearing 12 kinds of fruit, producing its fruit every month. The leaves of the tree are for healing the nations." Revelation 22:2

We may struggle here in a fallen world to obtain the best medicine as we would like, but I am glad someday, there will be an abundance made readily available for the nations in the form of God's good food. And so, until then, my honest suggestion is, eat as clean as your paycheck will allow. I know what it is like to struggle from paycheck to paycheck. I have more than once put food back that I just could not justify financially. So, at the end of the day, we strive for improvement, not perfection. Instead of processed, frozen and breaded chicken nuggets, go for canned chicken. Instead of fresh, organic fruits and vegetables in the produce isle, go for the frozen variety in the freezer section. Small, intentional swaps can improve your grocery budget while at the same time, improving your overall health. Minimize, to the greatest extent, the amount of hands through which your food has passed. This will cut out most processed and fake food, leaving you with the best, choicest food made available to invest in your health.

Listen to your doctor. No, not the guy in the white coat.

We have become blindingly trusting of any man or woman with "Dr." spelled before their name. We tell them our symptoms. We allow them to poke and prod all over our body without question. Heck, we will pay them money to tell us we are fat and out of shape, and get mad if we hear the same thing from our spouse! Then, we accept what they tell us as Gospel truth and embrace whatever script they fill out without question. We will run to the pharmacy, pay more money to purchase a product whose name is unpronounceable, and who's risks of side effects often outweigh the claims of the drug. Now, again, I am not demeaning doctors and pharmacists. I am demeaning our attitude and willingness to give up so quickly on our own health to leave it all in the hands of another person. These are our bodies. These bodies have been created to speak to us and be the first to clue us in on what is wrong. However, we have lost the connection to listening to our own body. Our body is our first doctor. It tells us every day if something is good or bad. It gives us signs, symptoms, and prescriptions for better health. It is time that we start to make an appointment to see this doctor again.

I am amazed at doctors' ability to identify an illness in a patient. I love diagnostic medicine. My most respected doctor in the world, though, has got to be a veterinarian. Consider the fact that these doctors are diagnosing patients who can't verbally speak and tell them where it hurts. The doctors have to figure things out in an animal that has no way of communicating the way we humans can. Have you ever noticed the first thing a vet asks the pet's owner? "What have you been feeding him?" Interesting, huh? Even more interesting is often their next step. A stool sample. They retrieve a small sample of feces and look to see what is going on inside of this poor animal, because a vet knows, the clue is in the poo!

This is just one way we can make an appointment with our own doctor. Our food goes through the exact same process every day of our lives. Nothing about the process of ingestion, digestion, and elimination changes from birth to death. Food goes in the mouth, breaks down in the stomach, is absorbed in the intestines, and then eliminated through the colon and rectum...clockwork. However, bathroom habits and signs point to an array of symptoms. You should know what to look for.

The Bristol Stool Chart is an easy tool to use to help identify some easily noticeable problems going on in the body.

BRISTOL STOOL CHART

	Type	Description	Condition
	Type 1	Separate hard lumps	SEVERE CONSTIPATION
	Type 2	Lumpy and sausage like	MILD CONSTIPATION
	Type 3	A sausage shape with cracks in the surface	NORMAL
	Type 4	Like a smooth, soft sausage or snake	NORMAL
	Type 5	Soft blobs with clear-cut edges	LACKING FIBRE
	Type 6	Mushy consistency with ragged edges	MILD DIARRHEA
	Type 7	Liquid consistency with no solid pieces	SEVERE DIARRHEA

Color is another determining factor that something could be wrong.

Stool colors

Brown stools: Having brown stools is normal and a sign of digestive health.

Green stools: Are normal after you eat spinach, parsely and green foods, but also a sign of a fast intestinal transit time.

Red stools: Concern for active bleeding in the digestive system (colon). May be caused by eating red foods (ex: beets).

Grey stools: Abnormal, caused by antacids, diarrhea medicines, heavy metals, bile, liver, pancreas problems.

White, clay-color stools: Too much rice, refined cereals, potatoes, bile, liver or pancreas problems, medicine, malabsorption problems.

Yellow stools: Too many fats, celiac disease, malabsorption problems. Sometimes normal when you eat only vegetables for a few days in a row.

Black stools: Tar-colored stools indicate significant gastrointestinal bleeding, concern for cancer or ulcers, too much iron from supplements.

Orange stools: Possibly caused by foods rich in carotenes (carrots, pumpkin, apricots, sweet potatoes) or products rich in orange food coloring.

Two-color stools: Fused together, first part is darker brown, second part is light brown or yellow-brown. Normal, a sign of being slightly constipated (old and new poop).

©natureword.com

The Bristol stool chart is not a diagnosis, but it may help to know when something is off, or to let you know it's time to make a call into your doctor's office.

The body has ways of telling us that something is wrong, and we can either save a trip to the doctor or know when it is time to go. For instance, if you are experiencing muscle cramps at night while in bed, you are probably deficient in potassium. If your muscles cramp while you are active, it could be a deficiency in magnesium.

Food cravings are another way the body tells us that something is off. A food craving is a sudden, insatiable desire to eat a specific food that doesn't go away until you have consumed that food. The cause of food cravings can be brought on by hormone imbalances, nutrient deficiencies, or stress. An often-hypothesized reason for cravings is that the body is simply craving a food that is rich in a specific nutrient that is lacking. It is the body's innate intelligence at work, sending you a diagnosis and prescription. For instance, a severe craving for chocolate may be an indication that you are low in magnesium. Craving ice? Check for anemia and low iron levels. There's good reason mac-n-cheese is the number one voted comfort food. Those who crave cheese are probably actually craving an amino acid called L-tryptophan. This amino acid acts as a relaxant for the brain and body, providing a sensation of comfort and tranquility. You probably had a stressful day! Craving water? A no-brainer...you are dehydrated, and your body is letting you know. Still thirsty? Check your insulin. Excess thirst and urination are the warning signs that your insulin levels are out of whack.

You have access to an amazing doctor and a plethora of medication, right at your very disposal. You will never have to wait around in a cold waiting room or stand in line for a mysterious little bottle of pills when you see this doctor. Your body is your first line of prevention and defense, and food is your easiest and most beneficial form of medicine. If we began to approach food as our pharmacy, we will see it in a whole new light. Your choices will become much more intentional and non-negotiable. You will see junk food as causes for disease and illness, and whole food as prevention and cures for them. And what's even better, you will FEEL the difference. Your body will respond to these choices. I believe after some time spent eating whole and clean, you will break some addictions, get rid of some inflammation, raise energy, improve sleep, and more. You will not want to go back to the old dirty way of eating. Let food be thy medicine and medicine be thy food.

With a Serving Dish

Up to this point we have approached food in several different ways, and nearly everyone has dealt with our relationship with God or with ourselves. I hope it has been eye opening for you. Food plays a vital role in how we connect or disconnect from God. It is fundamental to our own health and vitality as well. When we read the Bible, we see very quickly that there is a hierarchy of spiritual priority in our purpose for being. Our first priority should be obvious:

"He said to them, 'Love the Lord your God with all of your heart, with all your soul, and with all your mind.'" Matthew 22:37

Upon this command, Jesus said, hangs all of the law and the prophets. Our connection with food should always be approached in such a way as to honor, glorify, and connect us to the Lord.

And then, we must take care of our own fundamental needs. We wouldn't be physically capable of being present in the world if we didn't, right? When Jesus' disciples asked Him how they should pray, He honors the great commandment as the number one priority when He starts with,

"...Our Father in Heaven, Your name be honored as holy. Your kingdom come. Your will be done on earth as it is in heaven." Matthew 6:10

Then Jesus models the next priority, which is our own physical needs by praying,

"Give us today our daily bread." Matthew 6:11

Following this request, Jesus delves into our spiritual and relational needs with the Father,

"And forgive us our debts, as we also have forgiven our debtors. And do not bring us into temptation, but deliver us from the evil one. For Yours is the kingdom and the power and the glory forever. Amen." Matthew 6:12-13

End of the prayer, right? Sort of. Jesus adds a statement He felt needed to be addressed in order to have a healthy relationship with Himself,

"For if you forgive men their wrongdoing, your heavenly Father will forgive you as well. But if you don't forgive people, your Father will not forgive your wrongdoing." Matthew 6:14, 15

Jesus makes it clear that our relationship with others is vital to our own spiritual health and relationship with the Father. Of course, we must meet our own needs. Do you remember, however, the first and great command, to love God with all of your heart, mind, and soul? Well Jesus carried it forward and finishes His statement with,

"The second is like it: 'Love your neighbor as yourself.'" Matthew 22:39

And it isn't that upon only the first command hangs all the law and the prophets, but BOTH! You cannot have a right relationship with God without having a right relationship with people. So then, our hierarchy of priorities would be God first, our fundamental needs second, and people first. Wait. Two firsts? Yep. These are two sides of the same coin. You cannot have one without the other. To love God and love people is the fulfillment of all the law.

And so how does food play a role in that? Just as serving ourselves meets a fundamental need for our bodies, serving others meets both their physical needs, as well as our spiritual needs. What greater way to show love, mercy, forgiveness and grace than to share your meal with another person. In America, we have an entire holiday to commemorate this act. Thanksgiving reminds us of a time when our European ancestors were treated with life-saving kindness by the indigenous native Americans as they shared their food during the harsh wintery season and taught the pilgrims how to plant and reap in the new world.

Serving the Least of These

In the book of Matthew, Jesus explains the scene in the end times. He, the Son of Man comes in His glory and with His angels to judge and divide the sheep and the goats into two areas. The sheep represent the saved believers, while the goats represent the unsaved false believers. Verses 34-46 of chapter 25 record,

"Then the King will say to those on His right, 'Come, you who are blessed by My Father, inherit the kingdom prepared for you from the foundation of the world. For I was hungry and you gave Me something to eat; I was thirsty and you gave Me something to drink; I was a stranger and you took Me in; I was naked and you clothed Me; I was sick and you took care of Me; I was in prison and you visited Me.'

Then the righteous will answer Him, 'Lord, when did we see You hungry and feed You, or thirsty and give You something to drink? When did we see You a stranger and take You in, or without clothes and clothe You? When did we see You sick, or in prison, and visit You?'

And the King will answer them, 'I assure you: Whatever you did for one of the least of these brothers of Mine, you did for Me.' Then He will also say to those on the left, 'Depart from Me, you who are cursed, into the eternal fire prepared for the Devil and his angels! For I was hungry and you gave Me nothing to eat; I was thirsty and you gave Me nothing to drink; I was a stranger and you didn't take Me in; I was naked and you didn't clothe Me, sick and in prison and you didn't take care of Me.'

Then they too will answer, 'Lord, when did we see You hungry, or thirsty, or a stranger, or without clothes, or sick, or in prison, and not help You?'

Then He will answer them, 'I assure you: Whatever you did not do for one of the least of these, you did not do for Me either.'

And they will go away into eternal punishment, but the righteous into eternal life."

I believe a person is saved by grace, through faith in Jesus Christ, apart from works. I also believe that that kind of faith produces works. Here, we see the litmus given by Jesus to determine the righteous and the unrighteous is not a theological pop-quiz, but a "works evidence" test. Notice the very first test. "When I was hungry, you fed me. When I was thirsty, you gave me a drink." Feeding the "least of these" seems to be a pretty serious example of someone who has a right relationship with the Father. Jesus is essentially saying, "You both claim to be true followers but let me identify the real ones. Who here has fed the hungry? You? Alright, come stand over here beside me. The rest of you, you've been outed. To Hell with you." For you see, in feeding the "least of these," they were actually feeding Him. And what a way to show our love to Jesus than by feeding the poor, downtrodden, undeserving people that we see all around us.

It should take so much priority that we would be willing to sacrifice of ourselves to see to it. For example, I have known parents to go without so that their children might have what they need. Isaiah directs our attention to fasting. Fasting, as the prophet reminds us is to be done in order to break the bonds of wickedness. Hunger is certainly a bond of wickedness. And so, He says,

"Isn't the fast I choose: to break the chains of wickedness, to untie the ropes of the yoke, to set the oppressed free, and to tear off every yoke? Is it not to share your bread with the hungry, to bring the poor and homeless into your house, to clothe the naked when you see him, and not to ignore your own flesh and blood?" Isaiah 58:6, 7

There is hardly any kinder a gesture than to share your own food with the "least of these." Well who is the least of these? The obvious answer is the poor. The homeless. The hungry. It could, though, be the marginalized in your community. The person who you have held a grudge toward or who has hurt you. The person, perhaps, that you have overlooked for any reason. The pastor of the Jerusalem church, James wrote

"Pure and undefiled religion before our God and Father is this: to look after orphans and widows in their distress and to keep oneself unstained by the world." James 1:27

The responsibility of a parent or husband would have been to fulfill the necessity of food, but in the case of the orphan or widow, to whom does the responsibility fall? Ours.

I live in Asheville, North Carolina, which is an anomaly of the South. Tucked away in the Blue Ridge Mountains is a thriving artsy, hipster, outdoorsy community that loves music, food, and all things weird. It's a place that caters to the homeless population. It's a popular destination for a group of homeless called "travelers." Travelers choose to be homeless as a lifestyle. They hobo from train to train, hike into the city and set up residence in parks, alleys, or someone's couch. They typically don't approach anyone for handouts, and they travel in packs for protection and community. They are our least of these. You will find me, on a regular basis, hanging out at Prichard Park downtown, where the homeless gather during the day. It's not uncommon for me to spend time there, striking up conversations, praying for them, and taking them for coffee and/or lunch. That is the end of my motive. I'm not there to try to fix them or save them, just love them by feeding them.

We also serve a local ministry, aptly named, "The Least of These." They meet every Saturday morning downtown at 9am, rain, sleet, or snow. Every Saturday, hundreds of homeless venture out to get a hot breakfast served fresh and for free. We give them clothing and basic necessities, and pray with them. They are most grateful for the pancakes!

When it comes to using food to show love to people, keep in mind the quality of food you are serving. If Jesus came to our house for dinner, what would we feed Him? The same principle should be applied to others that we feed. Are we feeding them the canned goods that we don't like, or the food that has expired? Take not that you are doing your very best to provide wholesome, quality meals. Our church refuses to feed our little ones junk food. When we organize our annual summer youth program, we create a menu of food that is whole, real food. Things such as fresh fruit, celery and almond butter, grass-fed and GMO-free beef sticks. You might be surprised to hear this, but they absolutely love it!

We should be reminded how Jesus has exemplified this practice and attitude. For His first miracle, He turned water into the "best" wine. Twice He served thousands of people while in the wilderness loaves of bread and fish…and made sure there was plenty to go around. Before His crucifixion, He serves His disciples the holiest of meals, and shares His cup. After His resurrection and seeing His disciples have toiled all night fishing with dismal catch, He broils fish for them. And one day, He will spread out a banquet table for all of His followers to enjoy in His presence; a meal fit for a King of Kings.

Chapter 6

My Story, Part 2-After

The night that I collapsed on the bathroom floor, a severely broken man, was the final straw. My body and mind were completely wrecked. An auto-immune disease had nearly killed me. My adrenal glands were depleted to such an extent, I was unable to process even the smallest stress. This led to constant embarrassing anxiety attacks. My attempt at internalizing this stress took its toll on my spine. The tension twisted my lumbar vertebrae into scoliosis. Due to the lack of confidence I felt, my shoulders fell forward creating kyphosis, or "hunch back" in my thoracic vertebrae. My head fell forward in shame, putting extra strain on my cervical vertebrae and essentially losing my cervical curve. My entire spine was out of whack. Not to mention I had peaked at 225 pounds, a full 60 pounds heavier than my normal healthy weight.

As I write this, I am lounging on the 22nd floor of a luxury hotel in Chaing Mai, Thailand. I have flown half away around the world by invitation to teach on the subject of "Holistic Fitness" and "Optimal Rest and Recover" to a group of health and fitness coaches representing seventeen different nations. My life today stands in stark contrast to that of 2012.

Today, I am a master certified personal trainer. I have my own health coaching business that has taken me around the world and has brought those around the world to me. As a sought-after holistic health coach, I am seen as a nutrition and health expert and often find myself in speaking engagements and seminars. You can hear me weekly on my "Fit For The Kingdom" podcast where I deconstruct top Christian performers and distil down their practices in order to encourage and educate my audience in ways of optimizing their health so as not to compromise their spiritual health or their physical health. All this success can be greatly attributed to the destruction of my own health in years past, and also my re-construction following.

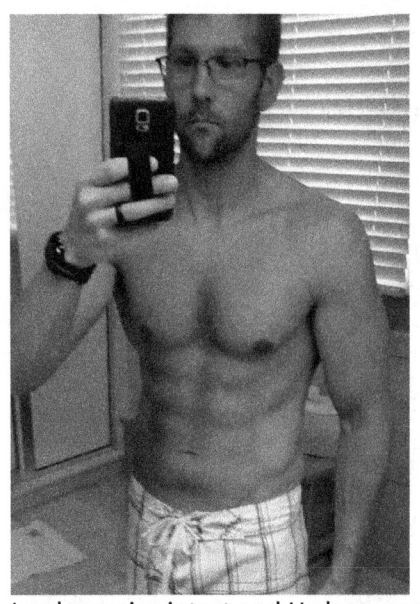

I have often claimed that the Trent prior to 2012 and the Trent following 2012 are two distinctly different human beings. The man that you would meet today is sixty pounds lighter and healthy. I have been able to lose this weight and keep it off. I have been able to straighten out my spine, relieve my back pain, and restore my adrenal glands. My depression is a thing of the past, too. My moods have leveled out and my outlook is optimistic. One of the most tremendous celebrations of health has been the remission of my autoimmune disease. My faith in the Lord remains intact and He has exercised His faithfulness over and over in my life to see a work of redemption and restoration. My blood work shows a very healthy individual physically, any my general disposition and responses to life give evidence of a healthy emotional individual.

So, how did this happen?

The road to recovery

Every person has a bottom. I'd hit my bottom and I realized it was either do or die. The entire duration of my darkened season, the Lord spoke to me through one verse. It was taken from a dialogue the Lord had with his disciple Peter. It was, in fact, a dialogue I believe He was having with me.

"Simon, Simon, look out! Satan has asked to sift you like wheat. But I have prayed for you that your faith may not fail. And you, when you have turned back, strengthen your brothers." Luke 22:31-34

I had felt the full-on assault from Satan. I knew what it was to be sifted. Sifting, however intended by the enemy, has a godly outcome for those whose faith remains intact. It acts as a purification process. I had been taken back to zero. All the impurities had been stripped away, and there was nowhere to go but up. It's a gift that allows a person to rebuild a burned down house. I'm going to share how I rebuilt my house. While I chronicle several avenues of reconstruction, I need you to hear this one thing. It couldn't have happened without changing my relationship with food. I will revisit that comment later and unpack it, but please pay attention to it.

1. The Spiritual Road

Though my spirit was broken, my faith was intact. I continued to call out to God day and night. I needed to hear His sweet voice. I needed to find out why I was so broken. I waited for a parting of the clouds and a voice from on high. As you might assume, that never came. I waited. I found comfort and a kinship to Jeremiah the prophet as he laid before the Lord a lament in chapter 3 of Lamentations.

"א Alef
1 I am the man who has seen affliction under the rod of God's wrath.
2 He has driven me away and forced me to walk
in darkness instead of light.
3 Yes, he repeatedly turns his hand
against me all day long.

ב Bet
4 He has worn away my flesh and skin;
he has broken my bones.
5 He has laid siege against me,
encircling me with bitterness and hardship.
6 He has made me dwell in darkness
like those who have been dead for ages.

ג Gimel
7 He has walled me in so I cannot get out;
he has weighed me down with chains.
8 Even when I cry out and plead for help,
he blocks out my prayer.
9 He has walled in my ways with blocks of stone;
he has made my paths crooked.

ד Daleth
10 He is a bear waiting in ambush,
a lion in hiding.
11 He forced me off my way and tore me to pieces;
he left me desolate.
12 He strung his bow
and set me as the target for his arrow.

ה He
13 He pierced my kidneys
with shafts from his quiver.
14 I am a laughingstock to all my people,
mocked by their songs all day long.
15 He filled me with bitterness,
satiated me with wormwood.

ו Waw
16 He ground my teeth with gravel
and made me cower in the dust.
17 I have been deprived[d] of peace;
I have forgotten what prosperity is.
18 Then I thought, "My future[e] is lost,
as well as my hope from the Lord."

ז Zayin
19 Remember my affliction and my homelessness,
the wormwood and the poison.
20 I continually remember them
and have become depressed."

Verses 1-20 not only spoke clearly how I felt, but it became my prayer. I reminded God often how I felt, and this passage said it perfectly. I know it sounds dismal, but I needed to be honest with God and let out my emotions. In response to my outcry, the Lord responded in the very same passage.

"ז *Zayin*
21 Yet I call this to mind,
and therefore I have hope:

ח Cheth
22 Because of the Lord's faithful love
we do not perish,
for his mercies never end.
23 They are new every morning;
great is your faithfulness!
24 I say, "The Lord is my portion,
therefore I will put my hope in him."

ט Teth
25 The Lord is good to those who wait for him,
to the person who seeks him.
26 It is good to wait quietly
for salvation from the Lord.
27 It is good for a man to bear the yoke
while he is still young.

י Yod
28 Let him sit alone and be silent,
for God has disciplined him.
29 Let him put his mouth in the dust—
perhaps there is still hope.
30 Let him offer his cheek
to the one who would strike him;
let him be filled with disgrace.

כ Kaph
31 For the Lord
will not reject us forever.
32 Even if he causes suffering,
he will show compassion
according to the abundance of his faithful love.
33 For he does not enjoy bringing affliction
or suffering on mankind."

My hope and waiting paid off. I had made an appointment to see my family physician to try to get some handle on my energy problems. After he read over my vitals, listened to by heart and breathing, and my explanation of how I felt, what he delivered as a prognosis left me stunned. "Trent," he said, "I believe you have lost your identity." "My identity?" I barked. The doctor replied, "You are eaten up with stress. You have put your identity into what you do. You have forgotten who you are. You aren't a pastor, that's what you do. You ARE a child of God!" His spiritual prognosis left me stunned. I wasn't sure what he meant. I was just interested in some quick fix to get my energy back! As I left, I chewed my lip as I pondered his words.

My next stop was the farm of a man who has been a vital part of my life and development of a holistic model of health. Jake Schwartz is an Amish herbalist. He and his son Samuel are trained practitioners in natural health modalities. They practice herbalism, applied kinesiology, iridology, reflexology, and a slew of other alternative practices. They have my full trust. I have witnessed their gifts of knowledge all my life, and experienced many cases of healing, myself. That day Sam was in, as Jake was at home still recovering from back surgery. I explained to Sam my symptoms. He tested me for everything under the sun and came up shaking his head. "I'm stumped." He said. "I can't see anything that's wrong, but I know there is. I think there's something else going on here." I sat, bewildered, with a feeling of losing hope. He continued, "On your way out, stop and see dad. Tell him what I said and get him to look at you." As we made our way up the gravel lane of their Indiana farm, we stopped the car in front of a modest little farmhouse, with clothes hanging on a clothesline flapping in the wind, and an old bearded man sitting on the front porch. I made my way to sit down beside him. "Jake, I just came from seeing Sam. He told me to stop and tell you that he couldn't find anything wrong." I explained. The old man, wincing at the pain from his recovering back pain, spun in his chair and began to examine me. Testing different muscles, glands and organs he sat back and began to offer a prognosis that left me astounded. "You're being spiritually afflicted." He said. "There is a demonic presence that is attacking you." I knew he was right. Continuing on he said, "You have lost your identity. You are working yourself to death and not resting in who you are. You have forgotten that you are a child of God."

With my back in so much pain, I had to bite the bullet and make an appointment to see a chiropractor. Dr. Bruce Cupp took x-rays and sat me down for an assessment. My spine was in terrible shape. Not only had I developed scoliosis from the internal stress, but my cervical spine had lost its curve and had begun to degenerate. In my sorrow and depression, I hung my head forward in shame. This prolonged depressed position had essentially changed the entire structure of my neck. Dr. Cupp began treatments to realign my spine and ease the pain. One particular day, while receiving therapy, I continued to share my outlook and feelings. With that, he asked me to stand and took me to a back room with a large mirror. Facing him, he said "Hold out your arm, and as I press it down, try to resist." I obliged. "You're strong." he said. "Now, turn and face the mirror and look at yourself. While you're looking at yourself, continue to resist while I push down." I resisted just the same, but this time I had no strength. My arm went weak. "That's so weird," I thought. He explained, "It seems to me, you have forgotten who you are. You are trying to manage all of this stress and you're putting it all into your body. You think you are a pastor. That's what you do. You have forgotten you are a child of God."

I couldn't deny these three affirmations. God was definitely speaking. Loud and clear. Using three men who didn't know one another, he spoke deep into my heart. He assured me, "You have forgotten yourself. You are not what you do. Pastor. Husband. Father. Church Planter. Yes, these are what you do, but that is not who you are. You are my child. You are loved. You don't have to perform for me to love you. There is nothing you can do, or not do, that will change how I love you because my love is not based on what you do. It's based on my relationship to you through my Son." In that moment of revelation, it was as if I had floated from the bottom of the deepest sea to surface and fill my lungs with a new fresh breath of life-giving air.

2. The Emotional Road

A man is not an island unto himself and I knew this. Yet I felt completely alone. I pushed people away without recognizing it. I alienated people that I loved and lost friends. Mandy had never dealt with these issues before and though she tried her best, she felt as if she was at a loss. She tried to take me away on a getaway vacation to the mountains. I was miserable there. I knew that I had to regain my sense of community and let people speak truth over me. I began by reaching out to mentors. Men who had poured into me in the past. To my surprise I kept hitting dead ends. The people that I expected to be there, for one reason or another weren't. I tried again. This time a friend who served as a full-time missionary in China. He suggested a man he was acquainted with who lived in Memphis Tennessee. He led a ministry that helped hurting pastors. To this day we have never met face to face, and honestly, I don't even remember his name! We corresponded over email the entire time. The reason I believe the Lord orchestrated such a relationship is that I don't think I would have listened to such hard questions as this man asked me. He could say anything he wanted, and it didn't matter. He didn't know me, and I didn't know him. He was able to be brutally honest and let me own it. If I didn't, it didn't affect him.

As he peeled away the layers of my rotten onion, we discovered how deep the rot went. I had to come to terms with my idolatry. I had made the work of ministry my god. I had to come to terms with my un-forgiveness. I had never forgiven myself for the loss of my brother, but, feeling that my unanswered prayers were a lack of my own faith. I had to come to terms with projecting my relationship with my earthly father which was based on "performance for pride" onto my Heavenly Father. I spent my childhood striving to make my dad proud to feel like I earned his love and pride for me. I knew I had been saved by grace through faith in Jesus Christ. That had been settled. Unfortunately, I had adopted a very false theology that taught, I could garner more appreciation from God and make Him proud of me if I could perform at a high level.

This man on the other end of the email suggested I read a book. I have to tell you I was in no mood for another self-help book from some emotional guru with all the answers. I decided to check it out and see what it was all about. I can honestly tell you; this book radically changed my life. It drove home the point I needed to hear and opened up an understanding that freed me from all the emotional turmoil that had been plaguing my soul. And I never read the first page. I'm sure it's a great book. I am not discrediting the author or the work inside. For me, the cover and title were enough. The book, "Jesus + nothing = everything". I stared at that title for days. It was as if it took everything that was weighing me down and lifted it right off me. I had been living a life that said "Jesus + (a good reputation)" or "Jesus + (a church this size)" or "Jesus + (this kind of success) = everything." I needed to know that Jesus + absolutely nothing else at all = everything! Jesus was my reputation. Jesus was my success. In Christ I was counted worthy and accepted. It was all clear now. Because I am IN Christ, I have the fullness of God in me. I needed nothing else to be satisfied. All my fulfillment could be found in Jesus Christ.

3. The Physical Road

As I lay in a hot tub of bath water soaking up the Epsom salt in hopes of relieving my chronic pain, I knew that something had to change in my physical lifestyle. Daily doses of 800mg Ibuprofen and hot soaks were not a means to an end. I had spent my life being "farm strong." That did not mean I was fit by any measure. I was carrying more weight than I had ever accumulated in my life, topping out at 225 pounds. I hadn't been active since my college days, when I tried to lift weights in the gym, having no idea what I was doing, or going on the occasional hike in the mountains. I had no cardio endurance to speak of. I wasn't even sure where to start.

One day with a little ambition I decided to try to go for a run. I didn't even own a pair of running shoes. I ran about a quarter of a mile and thought I was going to die. Not only was I out of breath and exhausted, but I developed the worst case of shin splints you could imagine. I hobbled around for the next week, swearing off running for the rest of my life. I couldn't even understand how someone could enjoy such an activity. Back to the bath soaks.

While hanging out in that bathtub, I began to research exercise. For some reason I needed to flood my brain and attention with images of fitness and workouts. It was so alien to me but keeping it in front of me provided some form of motivation. I surfed the web, navigating around topics such as fat loss, body building, weightlifting, and CrossFit. The idea of change began to prey upon my mind. It wasn't enough just to read about it, but I needed to ingest every bit of information that helped to educate me on the best, most efficient ways of getting into shape.

My first bout of exercise came under the coaching of a young man in our church who was a fitness enthusiast. Shaquille had battled his own health scares and turned his life around with diet and exercise. He was the closest thing to an expert as I knew, and he was willing to take me under his wing. Our city park served as the proving ground. When I showed up, Shaquille was waiting on me with a piece of paper. He had written a little program that involved 3 rounds of several bodyweight movements. Done at high intensity with short periods of rest, I had my first lesson in HIIT, or high intense interval training. Combining movements back to back like jumping jacks, squats, burpees, and lunges, it is designed to quickly shed fat and increase cardio endurance. It's also designed, I was convinced, to kill a guy like me. Shaquille made it look easy as we began. I gave it my best, and my best could not complete all three rounds. I was embarrassed. Unlike running, however, I refused to give up. This time was the last time I would give up.

I continued with Shaquille's workout program using bodyweight HIIT exercise. The first thirty pounds came off rather quickly. I couldn't believe the change I felt in by body to get so much weight off my frame. As summer came to an end, I lost the warm weather and sunny evenings. As the evenings grew cold and dark, I turned my attention to using the DVD led "P90x." Tony Horton of Beach Body became my new indoor coach. I began to take pictures of myself to stay motivated. It wasn't flattering pictures at this point, but I knew I would appreciate having "before" pictures to compare and contrast later.

I started at 225 pounds on a 5'9" frame. As the weeks fell away, so did my fat. My goal was to drop down to 180 pounds. I was amazed at how quickly I reached that goal. Time to set a new goal. 170 pounds seemed doable. It came and went. By the spring of 2013 I had reached 160 pounds. Six pounds lighter than my high school graduating weight. For the first time in my life I was sporting a six pack! I was really enjoying the results and the exercise that was responsible for them. As weather warmed, I decided to give running another try. I researched running shoes and ordered a pair from Amazon. Once again, I tried to run. This time, sixty pounds lighter and stronger gave me an advantage. I started with short distances, but each time I pushed myself a little harder and a little further. My lungs burned and my legs ached, but I continued. I added in weekly sessions of hill sprints to increase my aerobic capacity. Soon, one mile turned into two, then three, then four. Every day I put in miles.

That summer, our small town put on their annual small-town festival, "Sweet Owen Days." Every year to open the festival, the town hosts a 5k race. I had never run a foot race in my life! I signed up and showed up early. All I knew was to get out front quickly and stay there. I ran 3.2 miles of my best effort and came in first place in my age group. This win was what I needed to boost my confidence and give me an injection of unselfish pride to prove that I wasn't ruined. I could be rebuilt and improved upon. I repeated that win the following two years as well.

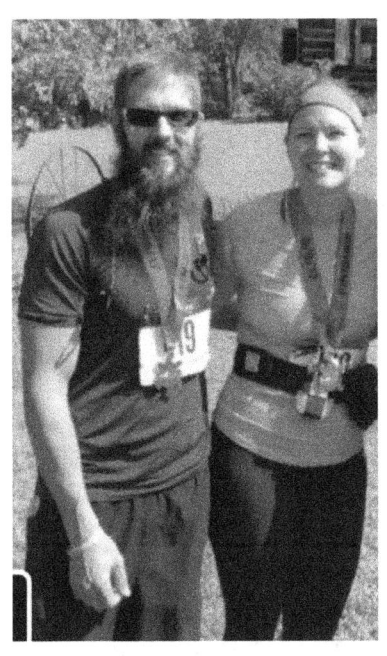My running improved and I began competing in half-marathons and trail running. My cardio was stellar, but little could be said for my strength. I had become skinny! I began to incorporate in CrossFit and fell in love with the performance aspect. With so much weight coming off, I had relieved some pain from my spine as well. It was time to build hard, solid strength and muscle gain. My friendship with Mark Bess became an investment in my health. Mark was an old school classically trained powerlifter. His basement was the ultimate gym. It was a "clang and bang" gym, outfitted with retired industrial workout equipment and tons of solid steel plates and dumbbells. I drooled at the opportunity to lift here. Mark became my master, and I his student. He worked with me and pushed me every day, teaching me form, technique, and motivation. He taught me the three major lifts, the bench press, deadlift and barbell squat. We worked incessantly on accessory lifts adding both, strength and muscle mass. We paid close attention to the deadlift. With my scoliosis and back pain, it was important to slowly build up strength and correction to my posterior chain. Weighing in at 160 pounds, I started lifting a modest 210-pound deadlift. With patience and consistency, I grew to pull a 405-pound deadlift and healed my scoliosis completely!

With exercise and fitness becoming such a passion of mine, having done so much to change my life, I felt it was time to give back. I started classes in personal training from the Federation of Professional Trainers. I wanted to give back. Jesus had prayed, not only for my un-compromising faith to endure, but that when I returned I would "strengthen the brethren." I received my certification in personal training and began training others to build their best physical selves possible. I started a gym called MasterFit and used that to train people to value their bodies because of their value to God. Later I became certified in sports nutrition and another certification in functional fitness, making me a master trainer. I began coaching nutrition and sports fueling at CrossFit Unbridled in Frankfort, Kentucky and went on to start my own on-line business, Trent Holbert Fitness. With this platform I could coach and consult clients all over the world. Geography couldn't hold me back any longer. Still, this wasn't enough. I needed to reach more people with the skills and education with which God had gifted me. I started the "Fit For The Kingdom" podcast, a platform that allowed me to reach the masses each week. My podcast takes lessons and insights from the world's top performers and deconstructs their practices in order to teach people how to live at such a level without compromising their physical health or their spiritual health, (just as I had had done).

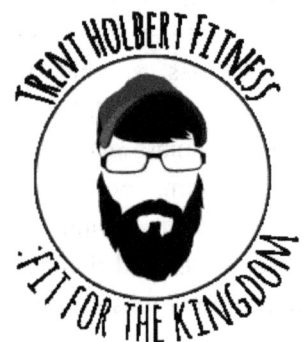 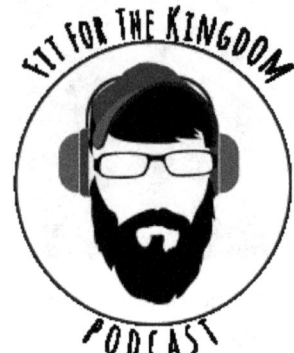

The Nutritional Highway

My journey to recover my spiritual health was vital to my recovery. No amount of attention given to my body would ever suffice if I didn't have a healthy relationship with God. My relationship with Him is the apex of health. With Him I have everything and without Him I have nothing. And my emotional health was a valid concern. In such depression I threatened my own life, my ministry, and the wellbeing of my family. I had to recover my emotional health and learn to value myself properly as well as to process stress appropriately. Though the Bible does say that physical health profits a little while spiritual health is more important (which is true), it doesn't say physical health in unimportant. As a matter of fact, the Apostle John shares his desire for physical with his friend and fellow laborer Gaius when he writes in 3 John 1:2, *"Dear friend, I pray that you may prosper in every way and be in good health physically just as you are spiritually."*

Physical health must have prominence in our lives, or else how would we transport our spirits and emotions to be present in this world? Yes, we are spirits, but our bodies give us the ability to exercise our spirits and present ourselves as living sacrifices unto the Lord. I believe in holistic health and having the balance of mind, body, and soul. My journey from total destruction, to total repair and total optimization was due to this fact. Each piece was vitally important, yet none of it would have come without a new relationship with food.

That may seem like an absurd statement. I'm not saying that any piece of recovery I used was unnecessary. I am saying, without a newfound respect for food and having a proper relationship with it, there would not have been these pieces applied for me recover. Let me explain.

As you have seen, food is essential and purposeful from the beginning in establishing a connection to God. As I considered my health, trying to get a game plan for how I might restore it, it occurred to me that what I had spent years practicing, to destroy it was my diet. I had such an unhealthy attitude toward food that, in return, that food made me unhealthy. I disregarded the value and importance of my own body. This was in correlation to my relationship with God. I didn't feel I deserved His love. I didn't feel valuable. I lived in shame and regret. My relationship with my Creator created the archetype for my relationship with food. "If I lack value and quality, then it doesn't matter what I eat." I thought. This created binge eating, and a disregard for quality nutritious food. My attitude toward food needed adjusting. Regardless of how I felt about me, I was created by God and for God. If that be the case, then what right did I have to treat it any less? Even though I had yet to find a healthy spiritual platitude, I held to what Scripture had to say was true.

I began to research food. Not diets. I researched how to eat whole foods. I started slowly, incorporating small steps. First, I stopped drinking calories. That immediately cut out sodas. With this one simple decision I began to see weight come off. I stuck to water, coffee, and green tea. I began to see food as fuel. Psalms 137:4 says that I was fearfully and wonderfully made. If I owned a brand-new Ferrari, I would not put an inferior fuel in it. So, why would I do that to a body that had been fearfully and wonderfully made by God? That caused me to make wiser choices with my food. Everything I put in my mouth would either work for me, or against me. I knew I needed to honor God by eating His food, in His packaging. That cut out all forms of fast food. It limited me to the endless supply of whole food. Delicious food. It helped to re-establish a connection with my creator, first through obedience, and then through gratitude and appreciation.

Now, wouldn't you know, once my diet changed due to a better relationship with the Lord and healing my spiritual self, my emotional health began to improve. I was eating clean, whole, and unprocessed food on a daily basis. Yes, it took time to shop and prepare my meals. Many people would argue they don't have the time. I would argue you do when you see it as a priority. I learned how to shop, navigating the grocery store to keep me out of the inferior sections of the market. Typically, that would be the center isles. Keeping myself around the parameter of the store kept me in the fresh produce, meat, and dairy areas guarded me from these places and ensured a cart full of whole foods. At home I found joy and took some pride in preparing my meals. I was the master chef of my kitchen and I could dictate what went into my food. I kept it simple. Choose a vegetable, a meat, and a fat. Then, bring it to life with spices. I fell in love with wild caught sockeye salmon and broccoli. So how does eating whole food change your emotional health?

The body essentially has two brains. It's true. You know about the brain inside of your skull. It is responsible for sending and receiving messages, holding on to memories, and exercising creative and logical thought. The gut does as well. Our second brain, the gut is a complex system that doesn't just digest food. It is a lifeline of health, both physically (digestion) and mentally (neurological).

Your gut is home to billions of bacteria that are responsible for turning on and off your genes. This is called "epigenetics." They are able to express your genes in ways that dictate your body's response to pleasure, stress, hunger, sleep, sex, and recovery. These bacteria need a healthy environment in order to feed and thrive to do their job. That environment is called a "biome." When your gut biome is unbalanced, your genetic expression can be thrown off quite terribly. The messages to the brain become damaged causing a myriad of health issues throughout the body. Oftentimes these problems are emotional.

Your gut is responsible for many neurochemicals related to mood. Serotonin is responsible for feelings of happiness and elation. Oxytocin is responsible for the feeling of love, both receiving and giving. Dopamine is responsible for pleasure. GABA is responsible for feeling calm and relaxed. These neurotransmitters are produced in the gut, and then sent to the brain to act up neuroreceptors. A bad gut biome will lead to bad bacterial health, which will lead to a down regulation in neurotransmitters, leading to apathy, depression, anxiety, and loneliness. Are you getting the picture?

Processed food is the leading culprit to bad gut health. Not only are we destroying our vital bacteria, but the very lining of the gut, itself. With an over acidic environment, oxidative stress from inflammatory foods, and chemicals in our food, we create tiny lesions in our gut lining causing "gut permeability." This "leaky" gut situation allows bacteria and toxins to pass through your gut wall into your bloodstream. This scenario can set you up for feelings of fatigue with aches and pains, and even disease.

Now that I began to eat natural whole food, my body began to heal itself. All my life I had a bad gut. I had suffered from gastrointestinal distress, nausea, and cramping. When I was small, I was skinny and gaunt. Later I lost control of my weight and couldn't seem to get it back. I never connected my gut health with my brain health. I noticed as my food choices improved by gut health improved. No more bloating and gas. No more cramping and nausea. And lo and behold, no more depression! My outlook began to change. Feeding my gut healthy pre- and pro-biotics (bacteria food) my neurochemicals and hormones began to heal. My thought pattern began to improve, and I felt pleasure again. My confidence grew to healthy levels! I began to feel superhuman. The effects were so astonishing that other people began to take notice. Without realizing it myself, I had stopped preaching using notes. After someone pointed it out to me by asking where my notes were, I realized by focus, clarity, cognition, memory recall and retention had all skyrocketed.

Emotionally I was in a place I had never been before. I never knew what healthy felt like until now. I had energy and ambition. My outlook had improved and so did my relationship with others, as it became more natural to show love and affection. I believe, now, heal the gut--heal the mind--heal the person! Food will always be your best anti-depressant.

My relationship with the Lord is healthy thanks much in part to food. My emotional health is at an all-time high, thanks to food. I couldn't neglect to mention my physical health. Without establishing a better relationship with food, what would my physical health be? I became passionate about health and fitness, and working out just became as normal to me as brushing my teeth. I valued by body and had the emotional outlook to drive me to improve myself. I enjoyed cross-training. I would go through a season of running, then switch to CrossFit or functional fitness. When I felt like it, I would spend time being a weightlifter and powerlifter. My body fat percentage dropped to a healthy range and my muscle mass skyrocketed. The food that I ate provided vital fuel to put in the hard work as well as the nutrients needed to reap the benefits. I learned the old saying is true, "you can't out work a bad diet." I also learned something new, that "abs are made in the kitchen." The better I ate, the less I needed to work out to stay trim and fit.

The most important aspect of my physical health, though, was the ability to play with my children. We could get down in the floor and wrestle without me giving up due to exhaustion and back pain. I had energy to take them for hikes and exploring. I was a dad that could finally be present in their lives. Playtime with them was important to me. So was the ability to protect them.

By the time I had regained my health, my two boys were around 7 and 9. We lived out in the country, far away from the dangers of the city and urban expanse. Nestled in the hills of Kentucky and near the end of a mile-long dead-end road, our house sat atop a ridge overlooking the Kentucky River Valley. It was a beautiful place to enjoy daily runs. About three quarters of a mile from my home was an apple and fruit orchard. My daily routine was to complete a morning fasted run to the orchard and back several times, accumulating between three to five miles a day. One summer day the boys wanted to explore the woods below our house with our dog, Jozi. My boys have been raised venturing around the woods and so this was common practice. I made sure my oldest son had a phone to call out in case there was an emergency. That day was the day I would get a call from him. Screaming and in a panic, he was pleading with me to come help. It was hard to make out what he was saying, yet I could put together clips and phrases, such as "there's another dog...its attacking Jozi…. there's blood everywhere." I was three quarters of a mile from our house. I turned and I sprinted. I sprinted the entire way, my lungs burning and my heart racing. I made it back to my house faster than I had ever ran in my life. I found my boys and our dog, shaken by an unprovoked attack from our neighbor's dog who had heard them down in the woods. Thankfully the injuries sustained were minor and the blood sprung from a nicked vein. The boys were unharmed, but still shaken and I was there to comfort them. Afterward, as the shock wore off, I meditated on this for a long time. "Before," I thought, "I would have never been able to run that distance, let alone be able to sprint it. Thank you, God, for my health and my ability to protect my family."

Performance, playtime, and protection were all factors in my relationship with food. My diet had afforded me a new lifestyle and a healthy family dynamic. There is one more aspect that I need to recount. Autoimmune diseases are incurable. Mine had tried time and time again to kill me. Hereditary Angioedema is a mutation in the H12 gene. This mutated gene causes my body to attack itself. I outlined this disorder in the previous section of my testimony, so you know what an ugly situation this is. Excruciating and deadly, there's no cure and no known cause. I was having an episode one to two times a month. Genes are funny. You're born with them and you can thank your parents for what you have. I was born with healthy genes. For some reason, I developed a SNP, or single-nucleotide polymorphism in my genes. We all have them. Small mutations that cause things from moles on the skin to diseases. You can't do anything to change the genes you're born with, or even the genes that mutate. However, you can change how your genes are expressed. Epigenetics is the science behind this activity. Genetic expression is a phenomenal way to take control of your genes and create a better situation. Oddly enough, I didn't even consider this. At that time, I had never heard of epigenetics or "dirty" genes. I was relegated to live a life of pain and fear of my autoimmune disease. When my diet changed, so did my genetic expression. The food that I was eating was healing my body, my gut bugs, and my hormones. Healthy food created healthy signals. My body went into full remission! I stopped having attacks and said goodbye to hereditary angioedema.

And to put icing on the cake, I stopped suffering from seasonal allergies and became impervious to poison oak and poison ivy rashes! I haven't been sick once since changing my diet. I previously suffered chronic sinus infections. I could set my watch to these infections. Every year for years, in the first part of November, I would suffer horrible sinus infections. They completely stopped. My acne on my back cleared up. I stopped getting cold sores. The aches and pains in my joints completely left. I felt like I was given a new body. A new life.

The Road Map

The first thing I did on my own after being born was to eat. That first meal was the absolute most important meal I could have ever been served. The colostrum, fats, and nutrients from that milk were engineered to safeguard me from sickness and develop my brain and body to become a strong human being. It was food, designed for health that God provided. Why do we assume that should end after we are weaned? He has provided life giving food for all stages of life. It is still available to us, but it is up to us to receive it.

Many people will come away from reading this with a better understanding of the importance of food. Many will have a desire to make a change to their diet and start eating better. Some will do it for spiritual reasons, others emotional or physical. Ideally all three. Then some will grow discouraged because they don't know where to start, or how to cook. My brother used to say about his cooking skills, "I'd burn a pot of water." Yes, you can tell someone of a glorious piece of land and describe all its wonders and beauty, but if you don't provide a map, they may never find it and enjoy it for themselves.

I want to leave you with some fresh, simple ideas for getting started eating better. These recipes are not gourmet, meaning they are not difficult or don't have too many ingredients to overwhelm you. I want to provide the simplest meals to get you started and hopefully you can pick up on the principles and start creating your own dishes.

Part Two:

Recipes
Frequently Asked Questions
Acknowledgments
References

Recipes

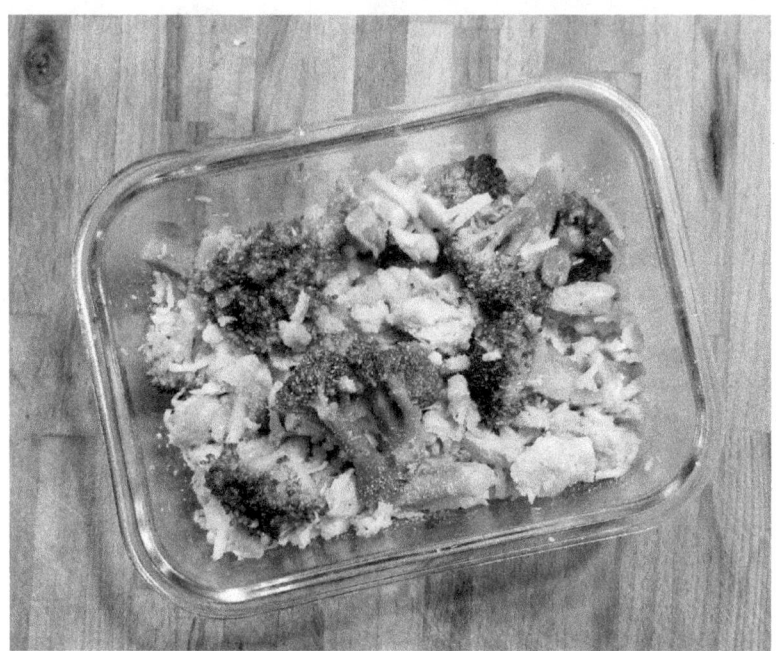

Chicken & Broccoli

1 (5oz) can white chicken
1 (12 oz) bag of steam broccoli
¼ Cup shredded mozzarella cheese
1 teaspoon olive oil
¼ teaspoon fine sea salt
¼ teaspoon crushed black pepper
Garnish to taste with Garlic powder, Paprika, Onion powder

1. Lightly brown chicken in a skillet
2. Steam broccoli in microwave
3. Add the two in a dish and mix in the olive oil
4. Add in the shredded cheese and spices.

This will provide enough for one meal. You can multiply these ingredients for meal prepping. For each yield, use a plastic freezer meal container and freeze until you are ready to eat.

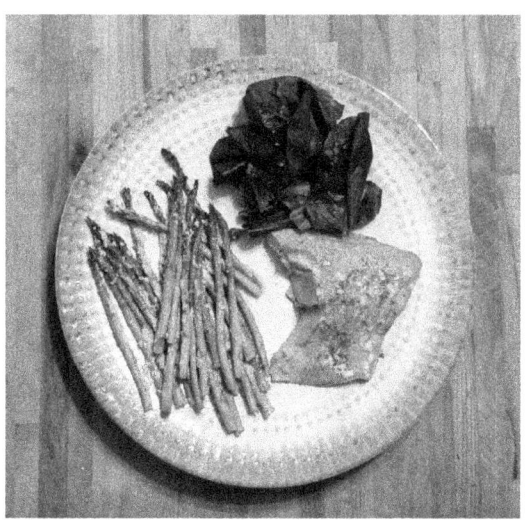

Salmon & Asparagus
1 (4-5 oz) Wild caught salmon filet
1 small bouquet of asparagus
¼ cup grated Parmesan cheese
2 Tablespoons olive oil
¼ teaspoon sea salt
¼ teaspoon dill
Garnish with Garlic, Turmeric, Purple Lettuce

1. Preheat 2 skillets with 1 tablespoon of olive oil each on medium low heat.
2. In one skillet add the salmon; make sure it is thoroughly thawed if it was frozen.
3. In one skillet add the asparagus.
4. Cook the salmon for 6-7 minutes on one side. While it's cooking, sprinkle the salt and dill (and turmeric and garlic).
5. Flip the salmon to allow finish cooking another 6-7 minutes or until thoroughly cooked throughout.
6. Keep the asparagus stirred until it becomes soft. Then add in the parmesan cheese. Allow the cheese to cook slightly into the asparagus, then remove from heat. Dash with sea salt.

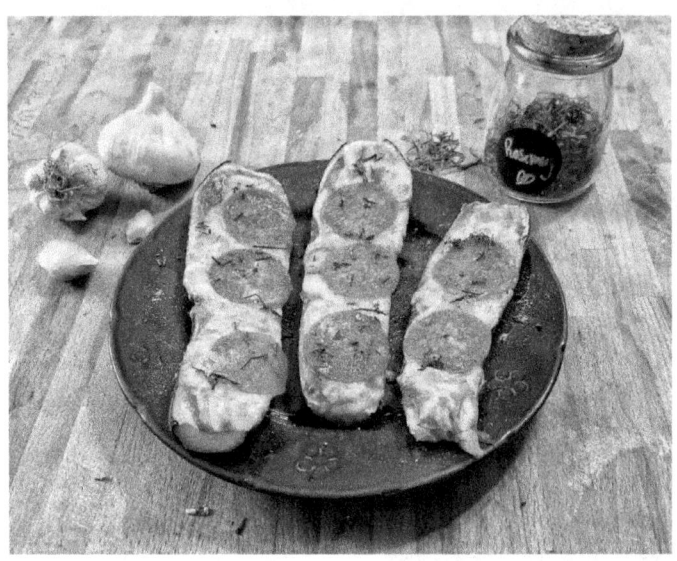

Zucchini Pizza Boats
2 medium sized zucchinis
½ cup shredded mozzarella cheese
4 slices of provolone cheese
¼ cup parmesan cheese
Thin sliced pepperoni
Garnish: Rosemary, Garlic, Oregano

1. Slice the zucchini in half long ways.
2. Spoon out the inside of each half.
3. Bake in a preheated oven at 400 degrees F for 25 minutes.
4. Add pizza sauce, mozzarella, provolone, and pepperoni.
5. Place back into the oven for another 5-10 minutes, or until cheese is thoroughly melted.
6. Garnish with parmesan cheese and rosemary, garlic and oregano.

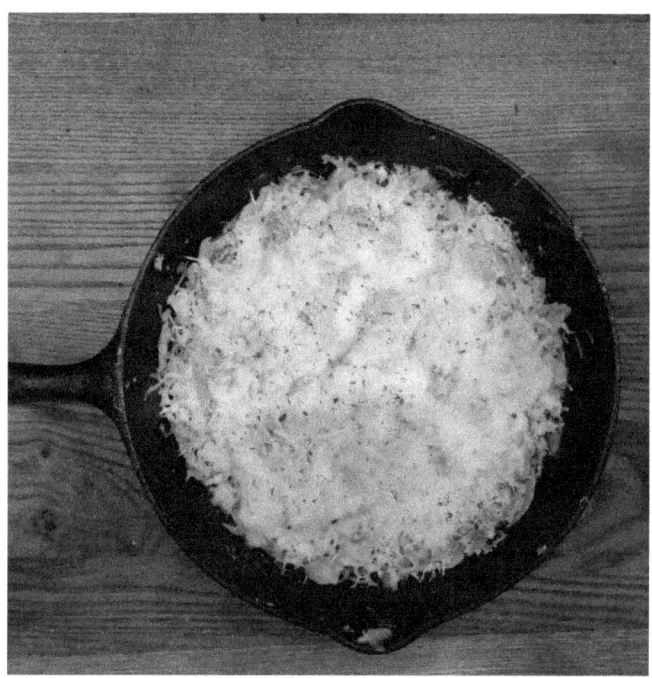

Easy Skillet Chicken Reuben

1 (5 oz.) can white chicken breast
Sauerkraut
½ cup shredded swiss cheese
½ cup shredded mozzarella
1 diced red bell pepper
½ cup thousand island dressing
1 Tablespoon olive oil
Garnish: Sea salt, Black Pepper

1. Heat olive oil in cast iron skillet over medium heat.
2. Lightly brown chicken.
3. Add in the sauerkraut and peppers and mix.
4. Drizzle over with thousand island dressing.
5. Cover with cheese and season with salt and pepper.
6. Serve when cheese is melted.

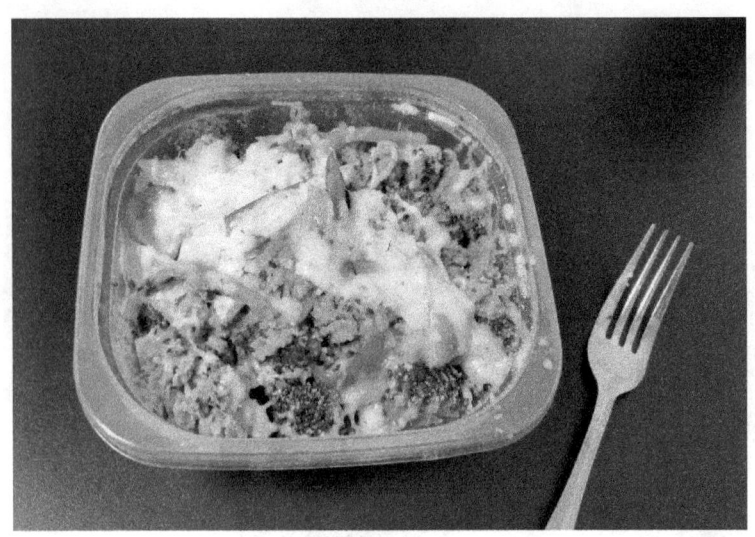

Italian Tuna
1 (4oz) can tuna
2 cups steamed broccoli
1 cup steamed assorted bell pepper slices
½ cup shredded mozzarella cheese
Garnish: Sea salt, Black pepper

1. In a skillet, mix and heat the tuna in the Italian dressing
2. Steam the broccoli and peppers and add to the tuna
3. Cover with mozzarella cheese
4. Dash with seal salt and pepper

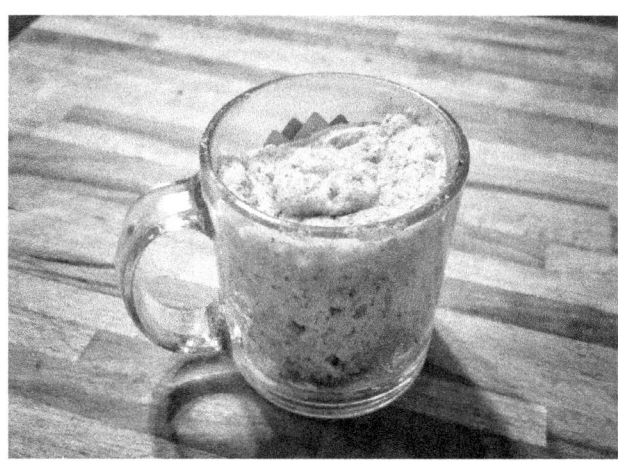

Mug Cake

2 Tablespoons almond flour
1 Teaspoon coconut flour
1 Teaspoon stevia
1 large egg
¼ teaspoon baking powder
2 Tablespoon unsweetened almond milk
Optional: Nut butter, Stevia sweetened chocolate chips, Coconut flakes

1. Mix all ingredients a coffee mug
2. Microwave 90 seconds

Frequently Asked Questions

1. Were Adam and Eve vegetarian?

The simple answer is yes, though the term or the idea would not have existed. When God created the earth and everything in it, He saw that it was good, and He blessed it. Adam was commissioned to be the earth's steward - to grow, harvest and enjoy all of God's wonderful garden. All except for the Tree of Knowledge. Death had not entered the scene until Adam and Eve sinned against God. Without the death of any animals, it would suffice it to say, all animals at first were vegetarian. The Bible tells us that "...sin entered the world through one man, and death through sin, in this way death spread to all men, because all sinned." Romans 5:12

2. When did people begin to eat meat?

Though we see death take place after the fall, it's not until Noah that we see animals become food. As God instructed Noah to gather "clean" and "unclean" animals onto the Ark, this was probably in preparation for a post-flood life. God then instructs Noah, saying, "Every creature that lives and moves will be food for you; as I gave the green plants, I have given you everything." Genesis 9:3. The practice of eating only vegetation was in accordance with God's original plan and probably carried out several hundred years after Adam's fall. We see Adam's son, Able tending a flock of sheep, however, in Genesis chapter 4. Some might assume this was for clothing, and most probably, religious sacrifice.

3. Should we be vegan/vegetarian?

We can see that God's original design for mankind was to live in peace with all animals, exempt from disease and death. Unfortunately, that ended when man rejected God's plan. God also created a design that allowed humans to enjoy public life without clothes! Much has changed since the original sin. Furthermore, much has changed post-flood. With the introduction of sin came the introduction of degraded epigenetics, meaning, our bodies are constantly degrading from our post-flood environment. The expression of our genes requires a new dietary system that is enhanced by the consumption of meat. Even our primal biology suggests that we are natural omnivores, with forward looking eyes, teeth for cutting and ripping, and an appetite and enjoyment for the taste of meat. It was God, mind you, who introduced meat as food. It was also God who gave the food laws regarding how to harvest animals as food. Jesus Christ is seen cooking fish over a fire. It's safe to say, we are omnivores, and what was pre-flood is a world we will not know this side of Heaven.

4. I like bacon and ham. Should we abide by the Jewish food laws of the Old Testament?

Though it has been argued since the first Gentile believers in the first century, it has also been laid to rest. There will always be legalists who continue to cling to Mount Zion rather than Mount Calvary. Food laws are a check list that keeps the legalist happy, though still damned. As previously taught, Kosher Laws were enacted in order to establish an identity in God. But, like the Feasts and Festivals, all are fulfilled in Christ. The manna that Moses gave has been fulfilled in Jesus Christ, the true Manna from Heaven. Our identity IS in food, i.e., Jesus Christ. The argument of Gentile believers who were pressured by Jews to continue Jewish tradition was laid to rest by James and the elders at Jerusalem in Acts 21, saying, "With regard to the Gentiles who have believed, we have written a letter containing our decision that they should keep themselves from food sacrificed to idols, from blood, from what is strangled, and from sexual immorality." That is the only food laws given to a believer. The Apostle Paul goes on to say in Romans 14, "For the kingdom of God is not eating and drinking, but righteousness, peace, and joy in the Holy Spirit. Whoever serves Christ in this way is acceptable to God and receives human approval. So then, let us pursue what promotes peace and what builds up one another. Do not tear down God's work because of food. Everything is clean." (verses 17-20a)

5. Jesus ate bread so how can it be bad?

We read about bread all throughout the Bible. It was a staple in ancient diet. Easy to make, easy to preserve, and easy to eat. Jesus was a fan of bread. He was born in Bethlehem, translated "house of bread." He called Himself the "Bread of Life." He instituted the ordinance of communion with bread, saying "take and eat." We can't get away with demonizing bread. We can, however, compare ancient bread and ancient lifestyle with today. If you could see the ingredients list of ancient bread you would see it was essentially organic, unrefined grain, salt, water, and yeast. That's it. Go to your local supermarket and study the ingredients list on the bag of a popular sandwich bread that the majority of Americans consume on a daily basis. Let me show you.

[Unbleached Enriched Flour (Wheat Flour, Malted Barley Flour, Niacin, Reduced Iron, Thiamin Mononitrate, Riboflavin, Folic Acid), Water, High Fructose Corn Syrup, Yeast, Contains 2% Or Less Of Each Of The Following: Calcium Carbonate, Soybean Oil, Wheat Gluten, Salt, Dough Conditioners (Contains One Or More Of The Following: Sodium Stearoyl, Lacitylate, Calcium Stearoyl Lactylate, Monoglycerides, Mono-And Diglycerides, Distilled Monoglycerides, Calcium Peroxide, Calcium Iodate, Datem, Ethoxylated Mono-And Diglycerides, Enzymes, Ascorbic Acid), Vinegar, Monocalcium Phosphate, Yeast Extract, Modified Corn Starch, Sucrose, Sugar, Soy Lecithin, Cholecalciferol (Vitamin D3), Soy Flour, Ammonium Sulfate, Calcium Sulfate, Calcium Propionate (To Retard Spoilage).] [1]

Are you sure you're eating bread? The "bread" that is manufactured has been stripped of its nutrients (literally) and then had nutrients added, or "enriched" back into it. Along with a nutrient swap comes an addictive food additive called sugar. And lots of it. Then comes a list of ingredients and words that you cannot pronounce nor know what they mean! Emulsifiers, fats, acids, and artificial ingredients. Have you ever noticed how quickly real bread will mold (about 3 days) in comparison to store bought bread (about 2 weeks). Something has changed in our bread since Jesus' day.

Another thing that has changed is lifestyle habits. Ancestrally speaking, people lived more active lives compared to our sedentary desk job lives. They could easily process the carbohydrates as energy without seeing the insulin spikes, crashes, and fat storage. Today, we don't have that luxury. While we are eating artificially enriched grains at every meal, we aren't working it off. And so, we can't demonize bread, but if we see it in light of today's standards and lifestyle changes, we can agree, it's best to minimize our intake and keep unhealthy ingredients out of our bodies, and insulin levels in check.

6. Will we eat in Heaven?

When we talk about what Heaven will be like, there is always some level of speculation. Scripture doesn't tell us everything we would like to know about this place. There is a great deal of mystery, however, there are some things that we can know or ascertain from what Scripture does teach us. It is not silent when it comes to diet.

The first thing, perhaps, that we need to consider is whether or not a resurrected body eats food. There would be no 'reason' to eat based on survival, and Revelations 7:16 tells us that in that state we will "no longer hunger or thirst." The idea here speaks, however, to going hungry or lacking. That doesn't mean we won't have the desire. Jesus said the one who hungers and thirsts after righteousness shall be filled. It's a desire. In Heaven, we are warranted many righteous and good desires that were always intended for us in an un-cursed environment. In John 21:10-15 we see a picture of a resurrected Christ preparing and enjoying breakfast with His disciples.

"'Bring some of the fish you've just caught,' Jesus told them. So Simon Peter got up and hauled the net ashore, full of large fish—153 of them. Even though there were so many, the net was not torn.

'Come and have breakfast,' Jesus told them. None of the disciples dared ask Him, 'Who are You?' because they knew it was the Lord. Jesus came, took the bread, and gave it to them. He did the same with the fish.

This was now the third time Jesus appeared to the disciples after He was raised from the dead."

Eating and dining in fellowship is such a beautiful, and good part of creation. It's most plausible to ascertain the Lord allowing us to enjoy this, for enjoyment sake and not survival.

Jesus' disciples believe they would dine with Him.

"When one of those who reclined at the table with Him heard these things, he said to Him, 'The one who will eat bread in the kingdom of God is blessed!'" Luke 14:15

And without lending any correction, the Lord affirms this assumption with a picture of the Kingdom,

"Then He told him: 'A man was giving a large banquet and invited many. At the time of the banquet, he sent his slave to tell those who were invited, 'Come, because everything is now ready.'

But without exception they all began to make excuses. The first one said to him, 'I have bought a field, and I must go out and see it. I ask you to excuse me.'

Another said, 'I have bought five yoke of oxen, and I'm going to try them out. I ask you to excuse me.'

And another said, 'I just got married, and therefore I'm unable to come.'

So the slave came back and reported these things to his master. Then in anger, the master of the house told his slave, 'Go out quickly into the streets and alleys of the city, and bring in here the poor, maimed, blind, and lame!'

'Master,' the slave said, 'what you ordered has been done, and there's still room.'

Then the master told the slave, 'Go out into the highways and lanes and make them come in, so that my house may be filled. For I tell you, not one of those men who were invited will enjoy my banquet!'" John 14:16-23

Jesus gives His disciples more hope during their last earthly meal together saying,

"I have fervently desired to eat this Passover with you before I suffer. For I tell you, I will not eat it again until it is fulfilled in the kingdom of God." Luke 22:18

In Revelation, John was commanded to write,

"...Those invited to the marriage feast of the Lamb are fortunate!..." Revelations 19:9

Or how about,

"The Lord of Hosts will prepare a feast for all the peoples on this mountain— a feast of aged wine, choice meat, finely aged wine." Isaiah 25:6

As I survey Scripture, I can see many examples and teachings of the idea of eating in my resurrected body. And some great benefits of eating in the age to come: no weight gain, food poisoning, cholesterol or diabetic issues! We get to enjoy the food of the table that has been prepared for us in the presence of our enemies. (Psalms 23:5a)

7. What will we eat in Heaven?

Scripture gives quite a tantalizing menu option for our appetites. Only two people have ever lived to taste food in its absolute purest form with perfect taste buds. As we gather together in a restored creation, we shall be satisfied at a banquet table. This time, not as guests, but as the bride! Can you imagine? A banquet of foods, perfect in every way!

-Ezekiel 47:12 offers us the best fruits and herbs.

-Isaiah 25:6 offers us the best wine.

-Revelation 2:17 provides "hidden manna".

-Revelation 22:2b gives us the Tree of Life that produces 12 different kinds of fruit!

In Heaven, we will eat perfect food. In Heaven, we will eat new food! In Heaven we will enjoy the tastes, sights, and smells of all the delicious food that is specifically grown and prepared for us.

8. Will there be meat?

My youngest son posed this question to me one day. To be honest, I had never given it much thought. "I sure hope so!" I exclaimed.

Some would say our diet will be in accordance with the pre-fall diet of fruits and vegetables. This would make sense, as the Lord restores all that was lost due to sin. Others would point to fact that to have meat would necessitate the death of animal. In Heaven there is no more death, so how could an animal give its life? These are very good observations that make good sense.

Could the Lord provide meat without having to kill animal? That seems absurd. Until, you realize He has already done this before.

"Then He commanded the crowds to sit down on the grass. He took the five loaves and the two fish, and looking up to heaven, He blessed them. He broke the loaves and gave them to the disciples, and the disciples gave them to the crowds. Everyone ate and was filled. Then they picked up 12 baskets full of leftover pieces! Now those who ate were about 5,000 men, besides women and children."
Matthew 14:19-21

Where did the thousands of extra fish come from for Jesus to fill the bellies of thousands of hungry people?

The prophet Ezekiel describes the new age as a place with swarms of fish in fresh river basins, with fisherman.

"Every kind of living creature that swarms will live wherever the river flows, and there will be a huge number of fish because this water goes there. Since the water will become fresh, there will be life everywhere the river goes. Fishermen will stand beside it from En-gedi to En-eglaim. These will become places where nets are spread out to dry. Their fish will consist of many different kinds, like the fish of the Mediterranean Sea." Ezekiel 47:9-19

Are we to assume that these fishermen were merely sport fisherman? Catch and release?

Or how about we revisit Isaiah 25:6 again,

"The Lord of Hosts will prepare a feast for all the peoples on this mountain— a feast of aged wine, choice meat, finely aged wine." Isaiah 25:6

I believe two things are possible as we look to our future home. One, there will absolutely be no death of any kind, for death shall be swallowed up and cast into the lake. (Revelation 20:14) And, two, we will enjoy the choicest meats! The Lord Himself will provide the barbeque and we will enjoy real meat by His hands of miracle and creation.

9. I have orthorexia. Can the Bible help me?

The last thing I would want to happen to you after reading this book is to develop any level of orthorexia. Orthorexia is a condition that consists of symptoms of extreme behavior due to the pursuit of a healthy diet. I believe, at times, I have suffered mild orthorexia. It can be difficult to pull back on the reigns of your diet when your goals are so committed. Many people suffer, as they constantly count every calorie, weigh out their food, and lose the enjoyment of eating. It becomes a life hindrance to say the least.

It doesn't have to be that way. The Bible offers help to the person who suffers orthorexia. I believe the root condition involves identity and pressure. At some point, our identity became skewed, and that misplaced picture of self, put an immense amount of pressure on us in order to keep up. Start by understanding what your identity is NOT. Your waistline does not define you.

The number on the scale is not who you are. Your muscles (or lack of) do not tell us who you are.

The Bible says in Psalms 139:14 that we "are fearfully and wonderfully made." That means, you have intrinsic value. That value is not based on your diet, nor is it based on your body composition. That value is given only by the One that created you. He made you to be you and declared you invaluable. How valuable? Value is dictated by the amount someone is willing to give for an item. God values you so much, that He gave His only Son, Jesus, to have you. That means, God gave the most valuable possession in existence in order to have you. That is invaluable. You are invaluable, just as you are.

You may look in the mirror and struggle with the image looking back at you. God sees you differently. Genesis 1:27 teaches us that we were created in the image of God. You reflect the glory and beauty of God, stitched together by His goodness, and reveled in by His tender mercies.

Our value and image are wrapped up in our identity. Not only were we fearfully and wonderfully made with intrinsic value and paid for with the most valuable commodity in existence, but that act gave us a new identity.

10. I have food addiction. Can the Bible help me?

Addiction is often associated with illicit drug use or some sinful behavior like pornography or gambling. Food addiction is by no means, less an addiction, nor any less harmful. Being addicted to anything is going to come with an assortment of problems. Food addiction can be linked to such health problems as obesity and diabetes. Emotionally it can contribute to shame and guilt. There are many reasons a person may become addicted to food, too. Do you stress eat? Many people find themselves eating without hunger. During stressful situations your body produces a hormone called cortisol. This stress regulating hormone causes an increase in hunger and many people find themselves craving carbs and fats.

Boredom eating will quickly lead to a food addiction. We may find ourselves hanging around the refrigerator or pantry when we aren't hungry at all. We're simply bored. And each time we reach for that snack out of boredom, we are essentially training the brain in a "Pavlovic" sort of way. Our brain becomes conditioned to want food anytime we get bored. The subconscious brain sends false signals based on behavior conditioning, not actual hunger.

Food addiction is as real addiction. In the same way that heroin addiction is an addiction. The brain isn't necessarily addicted to the substance, in this case, food. It's addicted to a little chemical produced by the brain called dopamine. Dopamine is a neurochemical that is responsible for the feeling of pleasure. Once it gets triggered, the brain wants it again, and more. Because the brain has the ability to remember what caused the dopamine response via the hippocampus, it craves that thing. Sugar is the biggest driver of food addiction for its power in eliciting a dopamine response.

The Bible can in fact help with food addiction. I will list what I believe are necessary steps for helping to break any food addiction, whether it is for specific foods or the act of eating.

- **Repent**

Repentance means to have a change of mind. It is an act or will to agree with God. When we chose food to comfort us or even pleasure us over and over again, we chose to deviate from God. Food and eating became an idol that took the place of God to be our comfort and pleasure. It's hard to admit, but the road to addiction is littered with idolatry. Spend time in prayer seeking the Lord's forgiveness for ever putting food before Him and choosing food over Him. Seek to cast down the idol of food and reconcile your relationship with God and food, putting each in their rightful place.

- **Fasting**

Addiction is bondage. It's an act that persists against your own will. As Jesus exclaimed, *"The spirit is willing, but the flesh is weak!"* (Matthew 26:41) Or, the Apostle Paul says, *"The things I want to do, I find myself not doing, and the things I don't want to do, I do. Oh wretched man that I am!"* (Romans 7:19, 24) This bondage is in need of being broken! Fasting has the ability to do this. Consider the prophet Isaiah,

"Isn't the fast I choose: To break the chains of wickedness, to untie the ropes of the yoke, to set the oppressed free, and to tear off every yoke?" Isaiah 58:6

Fasting is a powerful tool to break the bondage of food addiction. Spiritually speaking, it acts as an amplifier for prayer. You place yourself in a position to set aside time to pray, rather than eat. You pay more considerable attention to the specific need at hand, while communing with God and receiving His strength and healing. Fasting is also affective, physically speaking as well. It allows the brain to reset. It unplugs from the substance causing the dopamine response, and allows for new neuropathways to grow, rewiring the dopamine receptors. It's as if you are taking bad wiring, unplugging it, and then plugging it back in the right way.

- **The Word**

There is a reason you are reaching for food when you aren't hungry. There is a deeper, more pressing issue. Jesus, when tempted by Satan with food said, *"...Man must not live on bread alone, but on every word that comes from the mouth of God."* (Matthew 4:4). Ingest the Bread of Life. Reading scripture will allow God to speak more deeply into your life and touch the issues that are causing you to stumble. His word is truth and *"the truth shall set you free."* (John 8:32) People often approach scripture trying to interpret it and wanting it to say what they want it to say. I believe we are to approach scripture with humility and allow it to interpret us. The Bible can help break food addiction, if you go to the Bible for help.

Acknowledgments

My gratitude is a deep well to draw from and there are certainly not enough pages available to be able to list. As I can in no way take any credit for the ability to finish this work, my greatest thanks has to go my Lord Jesus Christ who is the true author and finisher of my life. He wrote my story and created in my heart the thesis which would become this book. I want to thank my amazing bride, Mandy. You have spent many years watching a very imperfect man grow, fail, and develop. My peaks and valleys have always been accompanied by your faithful love and support. Thank you to my parents, Tom and Judy, who instilled in me a love for God and His creation. Thank you for instilling in me a work ethic that refuses to give up, no matter the challenge. I want to thank the many, many mentors who have helped shape who I am as a man. And lastly, I want to thank you, the reader. You are the reason I have written this book. You were my motivation. May God bless you and keep you. May His face shine upon you.

References

Chapter 1: My Story, Part 1-Before
1 Genetic and Rare Disease Information Center, Hereditary Angioedema
https://rarediseases.info.nih.gov/diseases/5979/hereditary-angioedema

Chapter 2: The Beginning Plate (Food's Role in Establishing a Relationship With His People)
1 http://www.jewfaq.org/kashrut.htm, Tracey Rich

Chapter 5: The Believer's Plate (How Christians Should Approach Food)
1 World Health Organization, https://www.who.int/news-room/fact-sheets/detail/the-top-10-causes-of-death

2 Ben Greenfield "Fit For The Kingdom", Audio Blog Post. Episode 7: Ben Greenfield. Biohacking, Coffee Enemas, and Christianity. Trent Holbert, February 15th, 2017, https://podcasts.apple.com/us/podcast/ep-7-ben-greenfield-biohacking-coffee-enemas-christianity/id1195709802?i=1000381274947

3 Prescription Drug Spending in the U.S. Health Care System, American Academy of Actuaries, https://www.actuary.org/content/prescription-drug-spending-us-health-care-system

4 MedicineNet, "Top 10 Drugs Prescribed in the U.S." Omudhome Ogbru, PharmD
https://www.medicinenet.com/top_drugs_prescribed_in_the_us/views.htm

5 University of Rochester Medical Center, "A Guide To Common Medical Herbs"
https://www.urmc.rochester.edu/encyclopedia/content.aspx?contenttypeid=1&contentid=1169

6 The Bristol Stool Chart, https://simple.wikipedia.org/wiki/Bristol_stool_scale

7 Stool Colors: What They Mean, Marius Lixandru, March 13, 2018, https://www.natureword.com/stool-colors-what-they-mean/

Frequently Asked Questions
1 Fooducate, Wonder Classic White Bread, https://www.fooducate.com/product/Wonder-Classic-White-Bread/556190A2-32C7-11E3-A74D-1E047F0525AB

CPSIA information can be obtained
at www.ICGtesting.com
Printed in the USA
BVHW041213010320
573729BV00017B/637